Image-Guided Management of COVID-19 Lung Disease

Robert L. Bard

Editor

Image-Guided Management of COVID-19 Lung Disease

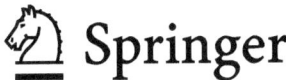 Springer

Editor
Robert L. Bard
Bard Cancer Center
New York, NY
USA

ISBN 978-3-030-66613-2   ISBN 978-3-030-66614-9   (eBook)
https://doi.org/10.1007/978-3-030-66614-9

This Springer imprint is published by the registered company Springer Nature Switzerland AG
The registered company address is: Gewerbestrasse 11, 6330 Cham, Switzerland

To my wife, Loreto, whose moral support during this pandemic generated the creation of this international collaboration and whose vision coalesced the advancement of noninvasive imaging.

Foreword

From the earliest reports of the novel virus SARS-CoV-2 causing a respiratory illness (COVID-19), clinicians remarked on the puzzling discordance between the degree of hypoxemia and relatively modest work of breathing observed. Early reports described this combination as "silent hypoxemia" and such patients as "happy hypoxemics." Similarly, soon after mechanical ventilation was instituted, unexpectedly high degrees of lung compliance in conjunction with severe hypoxemia was observed, attributed to an early phase "dry lung" with "hyperperfusion of gasless tissue" as opposed to the significant alveolar oedema and resulting hypoxic vasoconstriction observed in "traditional" acute respiratory distress syndrome (ARDS).

Next, an expert US radiology panel, after reviewing the first wave of CT scans of COVID-19 patients from Wuhan, reported in early March 2020 that the predominant finding was of an "organizing pattern of lung injury." This report, combined with our clinical recognition of the above clinical presentation (silent hypoxemia), led to our first impression that COVID-19 was presenting, in virtually all cases, consistent with a "viral-induced secondary organizing pneumonia" (OP) or its histologic variant "acute fibrinous organizing pneumonia" (AFOP). Viral-induced OP had been previously described in the prior severe acute respiratory syndrome (SARS), Middle East respiratory syndrome (MERS), and H1N1 viral pandemics. With SARS, OP and AFOP were reported in 30–60% of intensive care unit patients. However, the reported CT findings in COVID-19 suggested that secondary OP, AFOP, or both occurred even more frequently.

Although, both common and uncommon imaging patterns of OP have been described in approximately 60–90% of patients, the radiographic and CT findings are often so characteristic that they suggest the pattern of injury. The "archetypal imaging findings" refer to (1) peripheral, bilateral, lower lung predominant consolidation or even a frequent appearance in all lungs zones, and/or (2) peribronchovascular consolidation, which can extend to the subpleural regions in the lower lobes associated with patchy ground-glass opacities (GGO).

Although variable radiographic findings in AFOP have been described, patients who experience a rapidly progressive course exhibit imaging findings similar to diffuse alveolar damage (DAD), with diffuse but basilar-predominant consolidation and GGO. Those with a more subacute course may have similar radiological findings of cryptogenic OP with focal or diffuse parenchymal abnormalities.

Although our group, based on the combination of the clinical presentation and the characteristic findings of OP, concluded as early as May 2020 that early COVID-19 respiratory disease was primarily "SARS-CoV-2-induced secondary OP," our manuscript took months to publish given numerous rejections from prominent journals demanding either tissue biopsy (no center was performing lung biopsies in early COVID-19), and post-mortem findings all showed that OP had progressed to end stage DAD in almost all cases. Other reviewer requests were for randomized controlled trials showing that corticosteroids were effective in COVID-19. Thus, it was only after the RECOVERY trial established corticosteroids as the standard of care in the treatment of moderate to severe COVID-19 that our paper accepted for peer review and finally published in September 2020.

Despite this publication, secondary OP is still underrecognized as the underlying pathophysiology of early COVID-19. The importance that this knowledge becomes more widespread cannot be over-stated given that the increasingly adopted RECOVERY trial protocol (6 mg dexamethasone daily for up to 10 days) is insufficient in most patients with secondary OP. The reason for this is that it is well recognized among pulmonologists that secondary OP almost uniformly requires higher doses, prolonged durations of treatment, and a careful and monitored tapering given high risks of relapse when tapered off corticosteroids. Even more worrisome is that intensivists and hospitalists are unaware of the higher "pulse" doses traditionally required in the successful treatment of fulminant cases of OP or AFOP, a not uncommon presentation to the hospital or ICU.

With the belated realization that identifying the underlying pathophysiology and determining the correct treatment was largely apparent from the patterns seen on initial CTs, the importance of lung imaging in this disease cannot be overstated, with even more recent data showing imaging's importance in predicting need for monitoring and prognosis. Further, given the initial widespread, and still pervasive reluctance to send COVID-19 patients to CT scanning due to fears of contamination and spread of disease, this has led to an increased emphasis on utilizing imaging, largely with an emphasis on ultrasound and/or point of care. In synchrony with the evolution of treatment options, the numerous advantages of ultrasound, with its portability, ease of sterilization, and real-time diagnostics were appreciated.

The textbook compares and contrasts patterns of OP on CT with the latest in advanced sonography including high-resolution units, Doppler assessment of pulmonary disease, 3D histogram analysis, and venous imaging for thromboembolism evaluation. The input of multinational contributors adds to the depth of the material given the multiplicity of clinical findings continually emerging with the multifocal nature of this viral entity.

Front Line Covid-19 Critical Care Alliance   Pierre Kory
Palmyra, VA, USA

Acknowledgments

- Paul E. Marik, Pierre Kory, G. Umberto Meduri, Joseph Varon, Jose Iglesias, Keith Berkowitz, Howard Kornfeld, Fred Wagshul, Scott Mitchell, Eivind H. Vinjevoll, Klaus Lessnau, Emil Toma, Ralph Carter, Markus Hell, Giovanni Antonio Mereu, Mika Turkia, Puya Dehgani-Mobaraki, Brad Schneider, Gregory McNamara, Ginge Brien, Gregor Zasmeta, Miguel Antonatos, Jackie R. See, Patrick Jeanmougin, Tom Yarema, Morimasa Yagisawa, Ramesh Bolisetti, Curtis Crough, Andrew Hansen, Antonio Masciotra, Chris Newton, Annelies Moons, Rens Blommaert, Imco Flipse, Elena Panzer, Cathrien Bos
- … and, special thanks to my staff, Maryann Sta Rita and Aimee Arceo

Contents

Abbreviations

2019-nCoV	2019 Novel coronavirus
ADET	Italian Academy of Thoracic Ultrasound
COVID-19	Coronavirus disease 19
COVID-19	Coronavirus disease 2019
CT	Computed tomography
GGO	Ground-glass opacity
KD	Kawasaki disease
LUS	Lung ultrasound
MI	Mechanical index
MIS-C	Multisystem inflammatory syndrome in children
MODS	Multiple organ dysfunction syndrome
PIMS-TS	Pediatric inflammatory multisystem syndrome temporally associated with SARS-CoV-2
PMIS	Pediatric multisystem inflammatory syndrome
POCUS	Point-of-care ultrasound
RT-PCR	Reverse transcription-polymerase chain reaction
SARS	Severe acute respiratory syndrome
SARS-CoV-2	Severe acute respiratory syndrome coronavirus 2
SARS-CoV-2	Severe acute respiratory syndrome coronavirus 2
WHO	World Health Organization

Covid-19 Safety Protocols and Protection

Lennard M. Gettz and Robert L. Bard

1.1   Introduction

January 30, 2020—the World Health Organization declared a global health emergency due to the estimated 600 cases and 20 deaths from the SARS-CoV-2 outbreak allegedly spread from Wuhan, China to Taiwan, South Korea and a handful of cases in the United States. WHO reports indicated Italy, Germany, and France followed a month later with a significant spike of cases and deaths. Scientists reportedly have not seen a virus of this kind, but as the medical community tracked its origins and its geographic activity, the lethal nature of this virus showed the various ways that it attacks its host, its fast transmission and mutation rate [1–4].

Official announcement of a health pandemic in the U.S. arose by early to mid-February when the threat of this "foreign disease" became an American problem as states like California, Washington State and New York showed rising accounts of the virus. Institutions like schools and places of worship and soon followed all areas of commercial congregation areas like restaurants and shopping malls were ordered to close temporarily by local and state officials as an initiative of public safety.

L. M. Gettz (✉)
NY Cancer Resource Alliance, New York, NY, USA
e-mail: lg@321image.com

R. L. Bard
Bard Cancer Center, New York, NY, USA
e-mail: rbard@cancerscan.com

© The Author(s), under exclusive license to Springer Nature Switzerland AG 2021
R. L. Bard (ed.), *Image-Guided Management of COVID-19 Lung Disease*,
https://doi.org/10.1007/978-3-030-66614-9_1

1.2   Survivalism and the Global Demand for Disinfectants

By this time, national statements from health and government agencies widely reported that national public access to Covid-19 testing kits were significantly delayed [5], whereby major supply & distribution conflicts made the geographic accounting of cases impossible. The CDC and state officials announced public safety alerts to shelter in place, (self-quarantine), practice social distancing, conduct frequent hand washing and consistent use of face masks and face coverings. All this and other safety protocols became the new global routine from an "invisible enemy" that continued to increasingly infect our world population by the thousands each day.

By mid-March, reports showed the global economy was clearly impacted as the majority of industries suffered the significant downturn in consumer activity [6]. Meanwhile, as news headlines were focused mostly on the pandemic, industries directly related to managing our new health crisis received a major BOOM. This included communication technologies, PPE manufacturers, pharmaceuticals, and the sudden surge of sanitizing producers [7–9].

News reports of the March lockdown indicated widespread panic-shopping and premature hording frenzy, leading to empty shelves nationwide and a rise in desperate consumer activity. Brands old and new responded with a massive production campaign for disinfecting solutions. The War Powers Resolution Act has been said to help motivate new American suppliers and producers by expanding their product lines to include creating PPEs and other health and sanitizing products [10].

1.3   Fighting Back with Bacteria-Killing Solutions

The latest ruling of the U.S. Food and Drug Administration as of April, 2019 stated a final rule designed to help ensure that hand sanitizers available over-the-counter (OTC) are safe and effective for those who rely on them. "The rule established that certain active ingredients are not allowed to be used in OTC hand sanitizers, formally known as topical consumer antiseptic rub products, which are intended for use without water, that are marketed under the FDA's OTC Drug Review. The final rule also seeks to ensure that the agency's safety and effectiveness evaluations and determinations for consumer antiseptic rub active ingredients are consistent, up-to-date and appropriately reflect current scientific knowledge and increasing use patterns" [11].

Marketing sanitizers often used sell phrases like "Kills 99.9% of bacteria" on their products' labels describing antimicrobial, disinfecting, or antiseptic products. Others go deeper in their clinical descriptions with terms to reflect their scientific functions where the suffix "-cidal" implies the killing of something [12]:

– germicidal	– bactericidal	– fungicidal
– virucidal	– sporicidal	– tuberculocidal

Retail trends reported on the desperate consumer behaviors, including the erratic demand for any form of sanitizer. This product (among others) were identified to bring "a sense of security and a ray of hope for restoring personal health and safety." But for the discerning researcher, seeking out active ingredients in all products and comparing labels will find that *all sanitizers are NOT the same*. Some claim to "reduce" the number of germs, "kill on contact" or "prevent them from multiplying." A review of the required FDA's DRUG FACTS label on all sanitizing packages disclose the types of chemistries used, their concentrations, and safety instructions. They also include warnings of potential health risks that may leave uncertain lasting effects on humans or the environment.

1.3.1 Types of Antimicrobial Sanitizers

Antimicrobial sanitizers seen on the market fall into one of five base categories: alcohol, chlorine (bleach), phenol, quarternary amine, and quarternary amine + alcohol. These categories are usually aligned with one of the following active ingredients [13, 14]:

• Benzalkonium chloride	• Isopropyl alcohol
• Ethyl alcohol (ethanol)	• Sodium hypochlorite
• Didecyldimethylammonium chloride	• Ethanol
• Alkyl dimethyl benzyl ammonium saccharinate	

On a June 10 report, FDA.gov published that hand sanitizers using active ingredients other than alcohol (ethanol), isopropyl alcohol, or benzalkonium chloride are not legally marketed, and FDA recommends that consumers avoid their use. See www.fda.gov to review the latest legal status of these active ingredients listed [15, 16].

1.4 Commercial Sanitizing for Prevention and Maintenance

March–April, 2020. State, national, and worldwide agencies continue to track hospital cases vs. fatalities through the use of "curve diagrams" indicating the periods of rising numbers, the peak(s) and the patterns of decline of regional infection. This decline of cases (known as "flattening the curve") is credited by trackers and lawmakers on public response to the enforced preventive measures like isolation, social distancing and wearing masks. Without a vaccine or centralized treatment solution in sight, data on these curves collected only reflect the success of the quarantine and prevention protocols.

For all individuals, prevention included the battle against microbial contact and exposure and controlling our environment. This meant raising the level of cleaning practices to stricter measures like sanitizing, disinfecting and sterilizing of our homes and work areas.

According to estimates from the Centers for Disease Control and Prevention, one in 30+ U.S. hospital patients are known to acquire a minimum of one infection from a hospital stay. Healthcare-associated infections (HAIs) have been known to cause a significant number of permanent injuries and deaths to patients yearly, more than Aids, Cancer or auto fatalities [17].

The service industry reported a wave of cleaning companies emphasize "disinfecting services for Covid-19" for commercial, healthcare, and residential markets. These disinfecting service providers offer "hospital-grade" sanitizing solutions with EPA certified or regulated products and application protocols. Upon review of some of the top advertised service providers, certain products and sanitizing protocols are offered to manage HAI rates. These products are either "fogged" in enclosed spaces, sprayed with an "electrostatic applicator" or wiped on work surfaces. One common product is called Noroxycdiff—a hospital-grade, EPA registered disinfectant marketed commercially against SARS-CoV-2. The main active ingredient in our chemical is hydrogen peroxide [13]. Another is BIOCIDE 100, a product used for remediating mold. Meanwhile other companies offer applying VITAL OXIDE through an Electrostatic Sprayer or hospital-grade wipes [18].

1.4.1 Five Sanitizing Chemicals Identified Used in Hospitals [18, 19]

– Quaternary ammonium	– Hypochlorite
– Phenolics	– Peracetic acid
– Accelerated hydrogen peroxide	

1.4.2 Sterilants and High-Level Disinfectants [19]

1. Formaldehyde
2. Glutaraldehyde
3. Ortho-phthalaldehyde
4. Hydrogen peroxide
5. Peracetic acid
6. Hydrogen peroxide/peracetic acid combination
7. Sodium hypochlorite
8. Iodophors

Due to their strength and effectiveness as sterilizers or germ-killers, industrial disinfectants and sanitizing services are usually applied by trained professionals wearing complete protective gear. These chemicals often come with warning labels and possible health risks especially from misuse.

1.5   Personal Protective Equipment (PPE)

Prompted by the CoronaVirus outbreak, industry analysts indicated an explosion in response to the major demand for respirators and surgical masks, gloves, surgical gowns and all other PPE for all health responders in hospitals and private practices. By the early spring of 2020, Mayors, Governors and health officials nationwide began initiating mandates that anyone exposed to the public to wear protective masks or face coverings (ranging from scarves, bandanas to surgical masks) as an essential measure to prevent the spread of the Covid-19 contagion especially in Areas of Significant Community-Based Transmission. According to the CDC, members of the public are suggested to use simple cloth face coverings when in a public setting to slow the spread of the virus, since this will help people who may have the virus and do not know it from transmitting it to others. The CDC further stated that the best way to prevent illness is to avoid being exposed to this virus, however, it is always recommended that everyday preventive actions, such as hand washing and maintaining at least 6 ft of social distancing, to help prevent the spread of respiratory diseases [20].

Especially for the "front lines," the most widely publicized protective mask is the N-95 filtering face-piece respirators or FFP. it's five-stage-filtration design. Where surgical masks prevent contaminating others, the N-95 is an actual respirator filtering out 95% of the microbes and potentially hazardous airborne particulates like exhaust particles, pollen, dust, bacteria, and germs up to 2.5–0.5 microns. The Coronavirus' recorded size is 0.12 microns [21].

Due to the high demand for this respirator model, healthcare personnel sought out other products including foreign substitutes like the KN95. According to market sources, the KN95 is the "same product—as identified by the EPA when it comes to the 95% effectiveness of its triple micron filtration. 'N' means manufactured in the U.S. The USP code is K and 95 is China code. Then there's an AF94 from Korea and the FFP2 is the Euro code. They all have the same 94.6% rating with that 0.3 micron filtration" [22, 23].

These filtration masks are typically made of spun bound non-woven polyethylene built up one cylinder layer on top of another. Above that is a melt blown layer of polyethylene filtration, then on top of that is going to be another one of the spun bound polyethylene. Next is a PE wire, which is metal free, and that kind of holds everything together. Then on top, you have a cotton layer of filtration- the piece that goes across the face at the antimicrobial hypoallergenic piece of cotton. This gives you a decent feel to the face and the finishing piece on the mask [24].

1.6   Sanitizing with UVC Light

A rising trend in hospital disinfecting (as well as in commercial areas and public institutions) is the installation and use of UVC disinfecting technology. From small 8″ × 10″ boxes that extend the life of face masks in the healthcare field, to 8-ft. transportable setups that fully sanitize hospital recovery and surgical rooms, controlling infections with UVC is fast earning public acceptance as a low-risk, nonchemical solution with significantly proven effectiveness. Hospitals that use UV-light disinfection typically apply this technology as a second step to cleaning and disinfecting measures. This process is recognized by clinical infection control professionals and agencies to significantly mitigate infection risks associated with environmentally mediated transmission routes [25].

In 2006, the U.S. Environmental Protection Agency approved a test plan for Biological Inactivation Efficiency by HVAC In-Duct Ultraviolet Light Air Cleaners. The tests were conducted using three organisms, two bacteria (*Bacillus atrophaeus* and *Serratia marcescens*) and one bacterial virus (MS2). These organisms were selected because their sizes, shapes, and susceptibility to UV inactivation make them reasonable surrogates for biological warfare agents (BWAs). Generally, vegetative bacteria are readily killed and bacterial spores are more difficult. To model use in a VAC system, RTI used a test duct designed for testing filtration and inactivation efficiencies of aerosol, bioaerosol, and chemical challenges. The bioaerosol inactivation efficiencies calculated for the three organisms were 9% for B. atrophaeus, 99.96% for *S. marcescens* and 75% for MS2. The irradiance was measured as 1190 W/cm^2 at 161 cm (63 in.) upstream from the lamps with an airflow of 0.93 m^3/s (1970 cfm). The system had four lamps that were burned in for 100 h prior to measurements.

The concept of using UV lamps to inactivate airborne microorganisms has been an existing technology for many years. Much of the early work was directed at the control of very infectious microorganisms (particularly *Mycobacterium tuberculosis*, the causative agent of tuberculosis), often in medical facilities. Wavelengths within the short wave, or C band of UV-light (UVC), were found to be the most effective germicidal light wavelengths. UVC usually is generated by use of UVC fluorescent lamps. These lamps use electrical discharge through low-pressure mercury vapor enclosed in a glass tube that transmits UVC light (primarily at the mercury wavelength of 253.7 nm). Because this wavelength has been found to be about the optimum for killing microorganisms, UVC from mercury lamps also is referred to as UVG to indicate that it is germicidal. UVG has been shown to inactivate viruses, mycoplasma, bacteria, and fungi when used appropriately. (See the 2006 Test Evaluation Report by EPA [26]).

Due to the recent pandemic, companies developing this technology are (now) on the fast track to advance UVC installations for a wide range of professional and commercial environments. Specific testing is currently underway as to the efficacy against SARS-CoV-2 (the virus that causes COVID-19) but historically, UVC disinfecting systems worldwide have been tested and proven effective against pathogens that require even greater UVC dosages. "Every microorganism requires a specific UVC dosage for inactivation including the novel coronavirus. UV disinfection has been employed for decades in water treatment; these microwatt values have been used for reference to gauge UVC efficiency against a large cross-section of microorganisms. UV disinfection systems for room, surface & HVAC are (also) an ideal proactive measure to complement filtration"—stated UVC disinfectant firm Fresh-Aire UV.

1.6.1   History of UVC Applications

Niels Ryberg Finsen (1860–1904) was the first to employ UV rays in treating disease. He was awarded the Nobel Prize for Medicine in 1903 for his invention of the Finsen curative lamp, which was used successfully through the 1950s [27]. Updates in the technology for commercial use evolved as UVC germicidal lamps in the 1930s and have been primarily used in healthcare facilities. UVGI is highly recognized for addressing airborne microbial disease prevention (including influenza and tuberculosis). UVC is proven to prevent airborne transmission by deactivating airborne pathogens, but public use has been curtailed due to its potential to cause cancers and cataracts upon direct contact [28–30].

The history of UVGI air disinfection has been one of promise, disappointment, and rebirth. Investigations of the bactericidal effect of sunlight in the late nineteenth century planted the seed of air disinfection by UV radiation. First to nurture this seed was Richard L. Riley and his mentor William F. Wells, who both discovered the spread of airborne infection by droplet nuclei and demonstrated the ability of UVGI to prevent such spread. With the enduring research of Riley [31] and others, and an increase in tuberculosis (TB) during the 1980s, interest in UVGI was revitalized. With modern concerns regarding multi- and extensive drug-resistant TB, bioterrorism, influenza pandemics, and severe acute respiratory syndrome, interest in UVGI continues to grow. Research is ongoing, and there is much evidence on the efficacy of UVGI and the proper way to use it, though the technology has yet to fully mature.

Historically, investigations of the bactericidal effect of sunlight in the late-nineteenth century planted the seed of air disinfection by UV radiation. The first to nurture this concept was William F. Wells, who discovered the spread of airborne infection by droplet nuclei and demonstrated the ability of UVGI to prevent such spread. Despite early successes in applying UVGI, its use would soon wane due to a variety of reasons that will be discussed in this article. However, with the enduring research of Riley and others, and an increase in tuberculosis (TB) during the 1980s, interest in UVGI was revitalized. With modern concerns regarding multi- and extensive drug-resistant TB, bioterrorism, influenza pandemics, and severe acute respiratory syndrome, interest in UVGI continues to grow. Research is ongoing, and there is much evidence on the efficacy of UVGI and the proper way to use it, though the technology has yet to fully mature. An early study showed that NAIs caused a significant amount of biological decay of the bacterium *Serratia marcescens*. Exposure to NAIs showed inactivation or growth inhibition of the bacteria *E. coli*, *Candida albicans*, *Staphylococcus aureus*, *P. fluorescens* and has a lethal effect on starved *Pseudomonas veronii* cells. NAIs prevented 60% of tuberculosis (TB) infection and 51% of TB disease. Except for the inhibition effect of NAIs on bacteria, reports also showed that NAIs inhibited the growth of fungi and viruses [32] (Fig. 1.1).

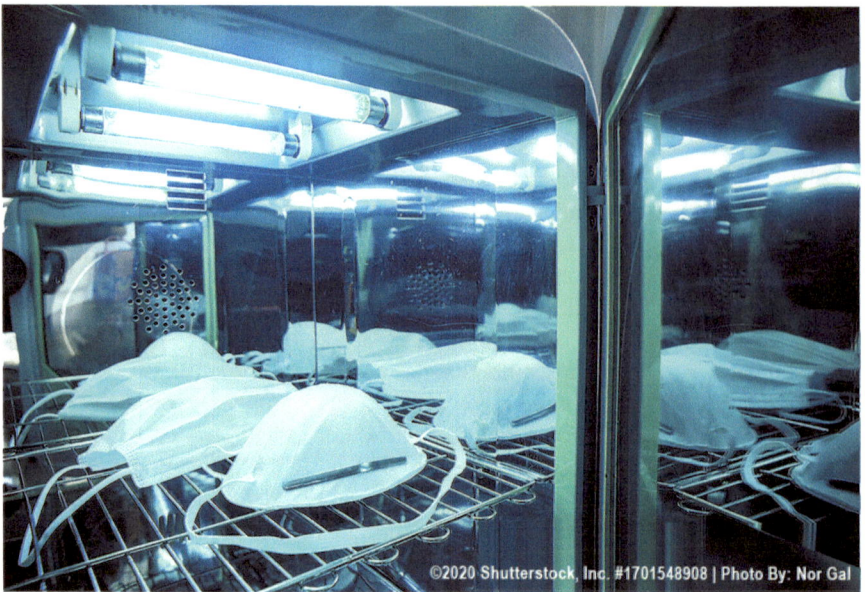

Fig. 1.1 UVC chamber disinfects used masks

1.7   Epilogue

By mid-June, the world has a recorded 7.9 Million Confirmed cases and 435,000 deaths from the CoronaVirus—with the United States leading at 2.18 M cases and 119,000 fatalities [2, 3]. New cases and fatalities continue to spike worldwide indicating its continued health threat and aggressive infection rates. State-run regulatory prevention measures proved to impact the case and mortality count while public recklessness reflects new spikes from this virus that continues to threaten our population at large. As the virus remains threatening the first line of defense will lie in modernized sanitization as the cornerstone of prevention (Fig. 1.2).

1.8   Summary

This chapter covers the market expansion of sanitizing products and technologies reflecting the current health crisis and the global demand for prevention and personal control of viral transmission. Presented are the active ingredients in liquid/sprayed disinfecting products, their efficacy and their antimicrobial strategy behind neutralizing the activity and spread of pathogens. In addition, the sanitizing industry also offers the innovation of UVC light to disinfect air (from airborne pathogens) and bacteria on surfaces. This historically tested innovation carries multiple applications dedicated to the immediate neutralization of viruses without the physical after-effects of chemical sprays.

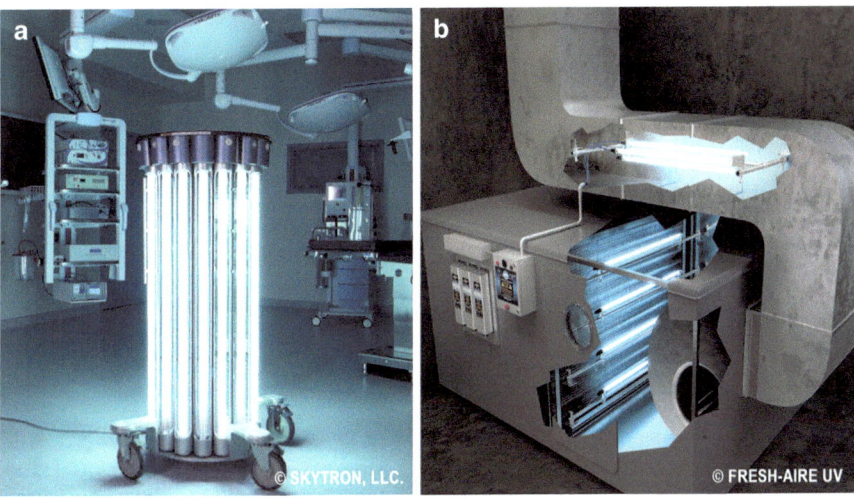

Fig. 1.2 (**a**) Operating room portable robotic sanitizer (**b**) commercial sanitizer used for hospital and industrial facilities situated in the ventilation system

References

1. WHO timeline—COVID-19 https://www.who.int/news-room/detail/27-04-2020-who-timeline %2D%2D-covid-19. Accessed 27 Apr 2020.
2. Google statistics: daily change Data. https://www.google.com/search?q=covid+cases+deaths +statistics&oq=covid+cases+deaths+statistics&aqs=chrome..69i57.8031j0j8&sourceid=chro me&ie=UTF-8. Source: Wikipedia. https://en.wikipedia.org/wiki/Template:COVID-19_pan-demic_data/United_States_medical_cases_by_state. Accessed 15 Mar 2020.
3. National Jewish Health. Stats coronavirus: information and resources. https://www.nation-aljewish.org/patients-visitors/patient-info/important-updates/coronavirus-information-and-resources/about-coronavirus-covid-19/current-coronavirus-stats. Accessed 15 Apr 2020.
4. Yale Medicine. 5 things everyone should know about the coronavirus outbreak. https://www. yalemedicine.org/stories/2019-novel-coronavirus/. 29 Jan 2020.
5. Harvard business review: why is the U.S. behind on coronavirus testing? https://hbr. org/2020/03/why-is-the-u-s-behind-on-coronavirus-testing. Accessed 30 Mar 2020.
6. International monetary fund: the great lockdown: worst economic downturn since the great depression. March 23, 2020. https://www.imf.org/en/News/Articles/2020/03/23/pr2098-imf-managing-director-statement-following-a-g20-ministerial-call-on-the-coronavirus-emergency Accessed 23 Mar 2020.
7. BusinessWire: Global hand sanitizer market 2020–2024. Evolving opportunities with 3M Co. and Godrej Consumer Products Ltd. Technavio. https://www.businesswire.com/ news/home/20200408005327/en/Global-Hand-Sanitizer-Market-2020-2024-Evolving-Opportunities. Accessed 8 Apr 2020.
8. PRNewswire/FinancialNewsMedia.com: demand for hand sanitizers still booming as FDA issues guidance on production. https://www.prnewswire.com/news-releases/demand-for-hand-sanitizers-still-booming-as-fda-issues-guidance-on-production-301074233.html. Accessed 11 June 2020.
9. Timeline of the COVID-19 pandemic in March 2020. https://en.wikipedia.org/wiki/Timeline_ of_the_COVID-19_pandemic_in_March_2020#1_March. Accessed 15 Apr 2020.

10. www.markey.senate.gov/—Senator markey calls on trump to use defense production act for massive wartime manufacturing mobilization for coronavirus tests, medical equipment (link). https://www.markey.senate.gov/news/press-releases/senator-markey-calls-on-trump-to-use-defense-production-act-for-massive-wartime-manufacturing-mobilization-for-coronavirus-tests-medical-equipment. Accessed 15 Mar 2020.
11. FDA issues final rule on safety and effectiveness of consumer hand sanitizers: https://www.fda.gov/news-events/press-announcements/fda-issues-final-rule-safety-and-effectiveness-consumer-hand-sanitizers. Accessed 11 Apr 2020.
12. Stanford Environmental Health and Safety. Comparing different disinfectants (link). https://ehs.stanford.edu/reference/comparing-different-disinfectants. Accessed 15 Mar 2020.
13. EPA.gov. List N: disinfectants for use against SARS-CoV-2 (COVID-19). https://www.epa.gov/pesticide-registration/list-n-disinfectants-use-against-sars-cov-2-covid-19. Accessed 14 Mar 2020.
14. A comparison of commonly used surface disinfectants. 2000. https://www.infectioncontroltoday.com/environmental-hygiene/comparison-commonly-used-surface-disinfectants. Accessed 15 Apr 2020.
15. FDA. Q&A for consumers: hand sanitizers and COVID-19—(link) https://www.fda.gov/drugs/information-drug-class/qa-consumers-hand-sanitizers-and-covid-19. Accessed 15 Mar 2020.
16. FDA.gov. Coronavirus disease 2019 (COVID-19)—(link) https://www.fda.gov/emergency-preparedness-and-response/counterterrorism-and-emerging-threats/coronavirus-disease-2019-covid-19. Accessed 14 Mar 2020.
17. CDC.gov. Healthcare-associated infections—(link) https://www.cdc.gov/hai/data/index.html Accessed 3/16/2020.
18. DEC.NY.GOV 7/17/2020—New York State registered disinfectants based on EPA list.https://www.dec.ny.gov/docs/materials_minerals_pdf/covid19.pdf. Accessed 17 July 2020.
19. https://www.hospitalmanagement.net/—"Top ten disinfectants to control HAIs" (link). 2012. https://www.hospitalmanagement.net/features/featureppc-disinfectants-hai-globaldata/#:~:text=4%20Hydrogen%20peroxide,the%20US%20FDA%20for%20sterilisation.%E2%80%9D. Accessed 15 Mar 2020.
20. CDC.gov. Factors associated with cloth face covering use among adults during the COVID-19 pandemic—United States, April and May 2020. https://www.cdc.gov/mmwr/volumes/69/wr/mm6928e3.htm?s_cid=mm6928e3_e. Accessed 15 Mar 2020.
21. FDA. "N95 respirators, surgical masks, and face masks"—https://www.fda.gov/medical-devices/personal-protective-equipment-infection-control/n95-respirators-surgical-masks-and-face-masks. Accessed 15 Mar 2020.
22. CDC.gov. Healthcare workers Ppe Faq-what is an N95 filtering facepiece respirator (FFR)? https://www.cdc.gov/coronavirus/2019-ncov/hcp/respirator-use-faq.html (Updated 8 Aug 2020). Accessed 1 Sep 2020.
23. Oklahoma State Department of Health: what should you know- KN95 RESPIRATOR. https://coronavirus.health.ok.gov/kn95s. Accessed 11 Apr 2020.
24. Honeywell. News/N95 masks explained. https://www.honeywell.com/en-us/newsroom/news/2020/03/n95-masks-explained. Accessed 11 Apr 2020.
25. CDC.gov. Ultraviolet germicidal irradiation - current best practices. 2008. https://www.cdc.gov/niosh/nioshtic-2/20034387.html. Accessed 15 Apr 2020.
26. EPA. Biological inactivation efficiency by HVAC in-duct ultraviolet light systems American ultraviolet corporation ACP-24/HO-4. 2006. https://cfpub.epa.gov/si/si_public_file_download.cfm?p_download_id=459522. Accessed 15 Apr 2020.
27. Nobel prize/Niels Ryberg Finsen- https://www.nobelprize.org/prizes/medicine/1903/finsen/biographical. Accessed 15 Apr 2020.
28. NCBI/US National Library of Medicine/NIH. The history of ultraviolet germicidal irradiation for air disinfection. 2010. https://www.ncbi.nlm.nih.gov/pmc/articles/PMC2789813/. Accessed 15 Apr 2020.
29. The history of ultraviolet germicidal irradiation for air disinfection. 2010. https://www.ncbi.nlm.nih.gov/pmc/articles/PMC2789813/. Accessed 15 Apr 2020.

30. Far-UVC light: a new tool to control the spread of airborne-mediated microbial diseases. 2018. https://www.ncbi.nlm.nih.gov/pmc/articles/PMC5807439/. Accessed 15 Apr 2020.
31. Johns Hopkins School of Public Health. The experiment that proved airborne disease transmission. How Richard Riley's findings about tuberculosis transmission inform our COVID-19 response today. https://www.jhsph.edu/covid-19/articles/the-experiment-that-proved-airborne-disease-transmission.html. Accessed 17 July 2020.
32. NIH. Negative air ions and their effects on human health and air quality improvement. 2018. https://www.ncbi.nlm.nih.gov/pmc/articles/PMC6213340/. Accessed 15 Apr 2020 (revised).

Robert L. Bard

2.1   Introduction

On December 31, 2019, the World Health Organization (WHO) was alerted to several cases of a respiratory illness of unknown causation emerging from Wuhan, China, and disease rapidly spreading elsewhere in China and abroad. Analysis of bronchoalveolar lavage fluid samples and electron microscopy revealed the culprit to be a coronavirus, a virus with a characteristic crownlike shape due to the presence of viral spike peplomers emanating from the viral envelope. On January 12, 2020, WHO temporarily named the virus 2019 novel coronavirus (2019-n-CoV) [1]. On February 10, 2020, the International Committee on Taxonomy of Viruses and WHO officially named the new coronavirus and the resulting illness severe acute respiratory syndrome coronavirus 2 (SARS-CoV-2) and coronavirus disease (COVID-19) [2, 3].

2.2   Covid-19 Pneumonia

COVID-19 pneumonia is a new, highly contagious disease outbreak with far-reaching public health, economic, and national security ramifications. According to current diagnostic criteria, laboratory examinations, such as swab tests, have become a standard and formative assessment for the diagnosis of SARS-CoV-2 infection [4–8]. Some patients with suspected COVID-19 pneumonia may have the virus detected by means of reverse transcription–polymerase chain reaction (RT-PCR) testing of the respiratory tract. However, RT-PCR is subject to false-negative results because it can easily be affected by multiple factors, such as

R. L. Bard (✉)
Bard Cancer Center, New York, NY, USA
e-mail: rbard@cancerscan.com

© The Author(s), under exclusive license to Springer Nature Switzerland AG 2021   13
R. L. Bard (ed.), *Image-Guided Management of COVID-19 Lung Disease*,
https://doi.org/10.1007/978-3-030-66614-9_2

insufficient cellular material for detection and improper extraction of nucleic acids from clinical materials. CT has a higher detection rate in patients with disease in the incubation period, especially for those with negative initial RT-PCR results. This finding showed that CT is helpful for early diagnosis, timely isolation, and treatment of COVID-19 pneumonia. For mass screening and real time results the Chinese and the Europeans quickly added lung ultrasound (LUS) to their diagnostic armamentarium. LUS has assumed a greater role as physicians gained more familiarity with the procedure and were able to efficiently multipurpose the imaging to the heart, liver, and kidneys. It is useful to analyze CT findings with the now widely available LUS data to better the pathophysiology of multiorgan inflammation. Since early reports based on chest radiography use words such as air space disease, infiltrates, pneumonia and patchy opacities, CT imaging has replaced the lower accuracy chest X-ray as the primary radiographic imaging tool.

2.3   CT Data Image Acquisition

Chest CT is performed with the patients in the supine position during end-inspiration without IV contrast administration using 1–3 mm slice thickness. Unenhanced CT images are evaluated in preset standard pulmonary (width, 1500–2000 HU; level, −450 to 600 HU) and mediastinal (width, 400 HU; level, 60 HU) windows. The following CT characteristics of the lesions were evaluated: distribution (left or right lung, single or multiple lobes, subpleural or peribronchial), attenuation (ground-glass opacities, consolidation), air bronchogram, vascular enlargement, interlobular septal thickening, mediastinal lymph adenopathy (defined as lymph node size ≥10 mm in short-axis dimension), pleural effusion, and pulmonary fibrosis.

2.3.1   Radiologic Findings

The subset of CT findings are ground-glass opacities (GGO), subpleural consolidation (Fig. 2.1a, b), reticular pattern and crazy paving pattern (Fig. 2.2a, b), air bronchograms and bronchial wall thickening (Fig. 2.3a, b), pleural thickening, subpleural lines, fibrous stripes and small vessel enlargement (Fig. 2.4a–d), air bubble sign, smooth or irregular nodules, and reversed halo sign (Fig. 2.5a–d).

Patients with COVID-19 pneumonia usually have ground-glass opacities (95%) and consolidation (72%). That ground-glass opacities were more common is similar to findings in previous studies [9–13]. Because of the highly homologous sequences between the genomes of SARS-CoV-2 and SARS-CoV [14], it has been speculated that the ground-glass opacities are caused by serous inflammatory exudation from the pulmonary alveoli and that the consolidation is caused by the increased inflammatory exudation. It has also been reported [15] that patients admitted to an ICU are more likely to have large areas of bilateral consolidation on CT scans, whereas

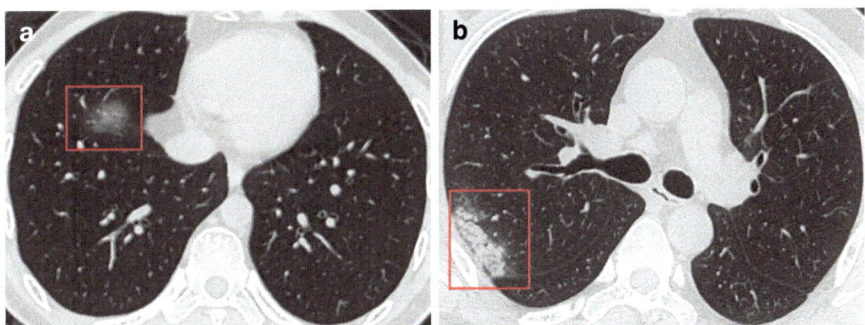

Fig. 2.1 (**a**) Ground-glass opacity (frame) (**b**) subpleural consolidation (frame). Eur Radiol 2020 30:4381 Zheng Ye with permission order#501589172

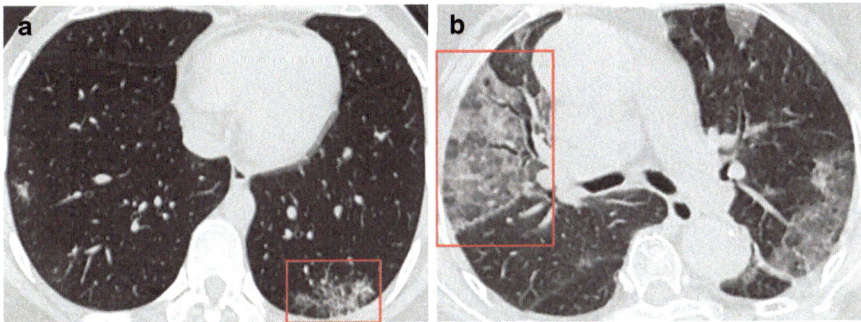

Fig. 2.2 (**a**) Reticular pattern (frame) (**b**) crazy paving pattern (frame). Eur Radiol 2020 30:4381 Zheng Ye with permission order#501589172

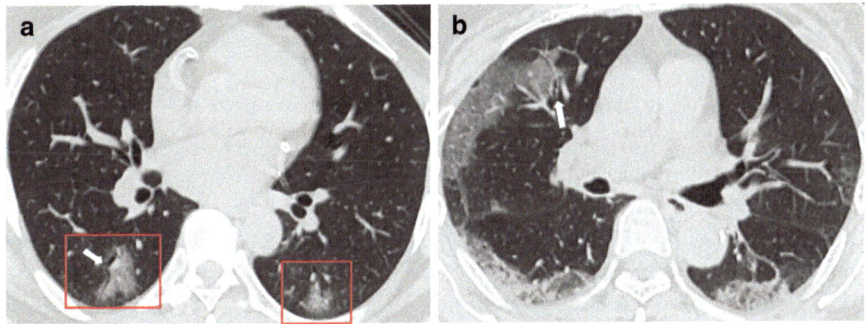

Fig. 2.3 (**a**) Air bronchogram sign with GGO (frame, arrow) (**b**) bronchial thickening (arrow). Eur Radiol 2020 30:4381 Zheng Ye with permission order#501589172

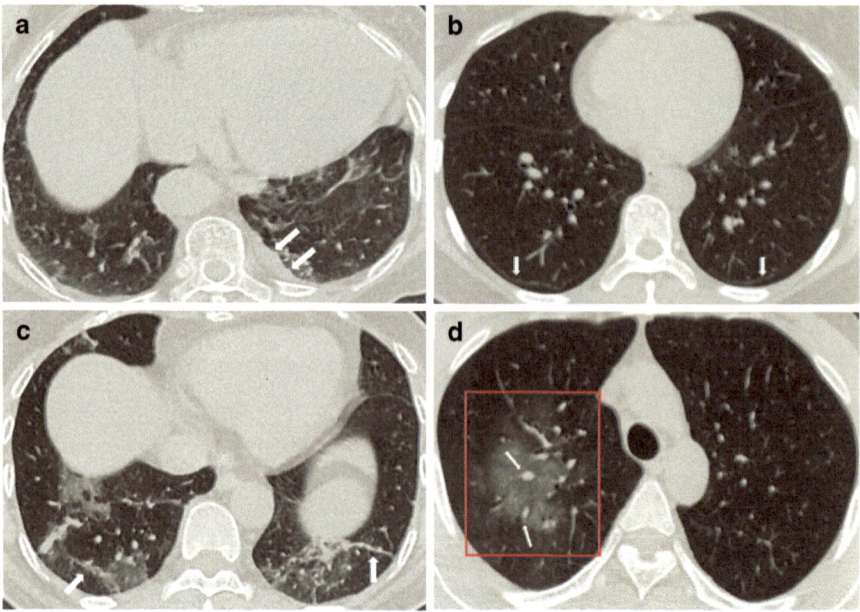

Fig. 2.4 (**a**) Pleural thickening (arrow) (**b**) subpleural lines (arrow) (**c**) fibrous stripes (arrow) (**d**) dilated vessels (arrows). Eur Radiol 2020 30:4381 Zheng Ye with permission order#501589172

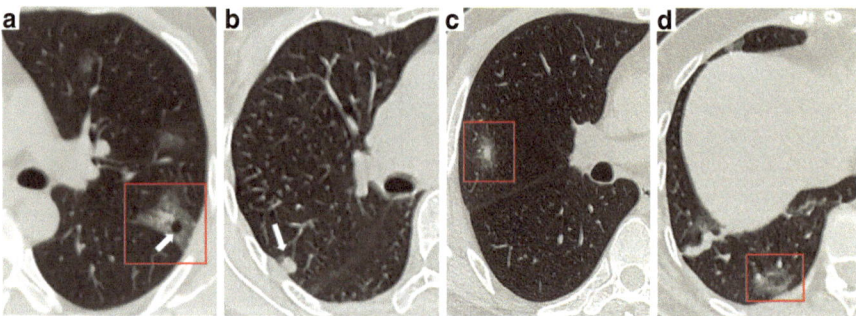

Fig. 2.5 (**a**) GGO with air bubble (frame) (**b**) irregular nodule (frame) (**c**) smooth nodule (frame) (**d**) reversed halo sign (frame). Eur Radiol 2020 30:4381 Zheng Ye with permission order#501589172

patients not needing admission and presenting with milder forms of the illness are more likely to have ground-glass opacities and small areas of consolidation. That is, the disease usually manifests ground-glass opacities in the early stage and then the area or areas of consolidation increase as the disease progresses, which may be predictive of severe complications, such as acute respiratory disease. Other CT features included air bronchogram, vascular enlargement, and interlobular septal

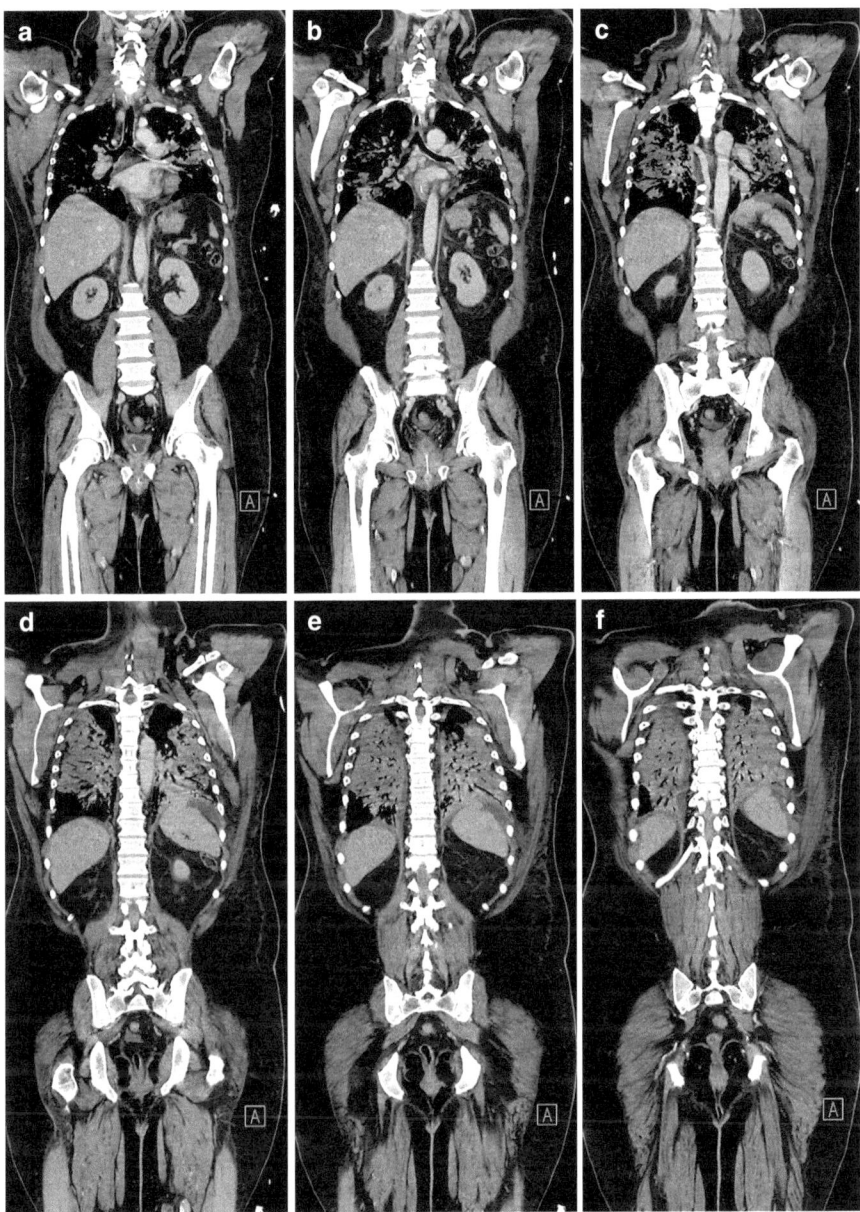

Fig. 2.6 (**a–f**) Whole body CT coronal scans demonstrate progression of pneumonic consolidation from anterior to posterior. Note progression of small consolidations to complete lobar pneumonia bilaterally. (Siemens Sequoia CT-Covid34—39 with permission)

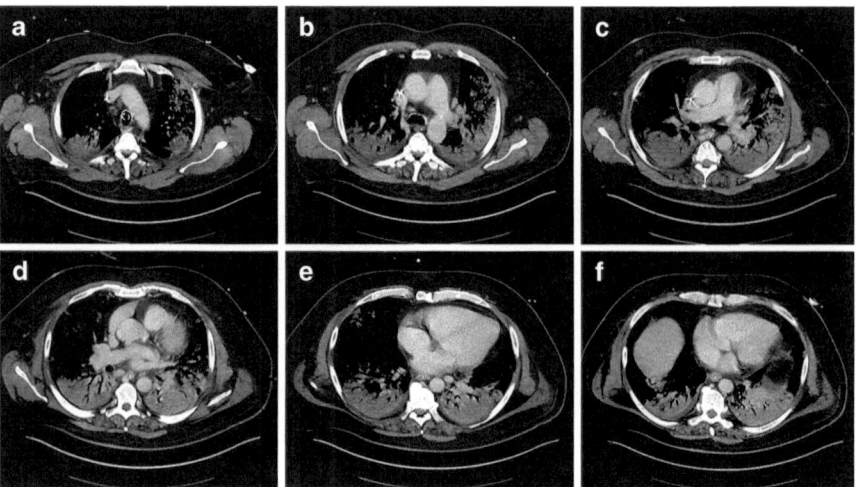

Fig. 2.7 (a–f) Sequential 1 cm slices of consolidation (Siemens Sequioa CT-Covid 40—45 with permission)

thickening. With superimposed ground-glass opacification, the interlobular septal thickening can form the crazy paving pattern. Pleural effusion is uncommon and may be related to the underlying diseases. Sequential frontal imaging on whole body CT shows the lungs, abdomen, neck, spine and axial skeleton since many organ systems may be involved (Fig. 2.6a–f) This may be combined with cross-sectional imaging (Fig. 2.7a–f) that is used for image guided treatments.

2.3.2   Early Clinical Course

We found that compared with the findings in patients with positive initial RT-PCR results, the area of consolidation lesions in the patients with negative initial RT-PCR results was smaller. In the group with negative initial RT-PCR results, most of the lesions appeared as ground-glass opacities or opacities mixed with a small area of consolidation, which indicated that the disease was in its early stage. A recent study [16] had a similar result: all five of the patients in the study had ground-glass opacification, and only two had mixed consolidation. It has been reported [15] that the presence of consolidation lesions suggests an organizing pneumonia pattern of lung injury. A small area of consolidation indicates that the injury to lung tissue is mild, increasing the possibility of negative initial RT-PCR results. In contrast, when the area of consolidation is large, the possibility of negative initial RT-PCR results decreases. Early specific signs of pneumonitis include vascular thickening, air bronchograms, crazy paving pattern (due to superimposed reticular and/or interlobular septal thickening and visible intralobular lines or overlay of ground-glass opacities with fibrosis or vascular thickening) and the halo sign surrounding the GGO that may represent early diffuse alveolar damage from cytokine storm edematous response. GGO is further subdivided into pure GGO and GGO with reticular and/or interlobular septal thickening. A variation on the GGO is termed the atoll sign (or reversed halo sign) where central lucency due to higher peripheral attenuation occurs and is generally later in the disease. In early disease pleural effusion, pleural thickening, peribronchovascular opacities, bronchiectasis and extrapulmonary findings such as enlargement of mediastinal and hilar lymph nodes are generally absent. As the disease has progressed over the past year there is an increasing incidence of post infection complications in survivors, notably traction bronchiectasis. This post inflammatory process may be due to peribronchial fibrosis that mechanically pulls the bronchial walls or bronchiolization of the bronchi from many causes.

2.3.3   Comparison with Influenza Pneumonia

CT manifestations of viral pneumonitis by similar viruses show common findings including GGO and consolidations. Most consolidative lesions in the pulmonary parenchyma in adult COVID 19 patients are located in the peripheral zones while influenza virus pneumonia tended to show mucoid impaction and pleural effusions. Mucoid impaction is generated by the fact that the influenza virus tends to affect both large and small airways (as well as the lung parenchyma) producing excessive mucus production. Histologic findings of aggressive pneumonia include membrane formation, diffuse alveolar damage, interstitial lymphocyte infiltration, airspace hemorrhage, edema, fibrin and type II cell proliferation [17, 18].

Apart from the typical CT findings of bilateral ground-glass opacities and consolidation, subpleural distribution was observed. The less pulmonary consolidation found at CT, the greater was the possibility of initial negative RT-PCR results [19]. Although CT is not the final standard for the diagnosis of COVID-19 pneumonia, it nevertheless plays an irreplaceable role. When patients with suspected COVID-19 pneumonia who have an epidemiologic history and typical CT features have negative initial RT-PCR results, repeated RT-PCR tests and patient isolation should be considered. Prognostication may be based on a CT scoring system based on time from disease progression to resolution and percentage of pulmonary parenchyma involved with Grade 1 less than 5% to Grade 5 more than 75% for the GGO, crazy paving pattern and consolidation. In critical cases where pulmonary emboli is suspect, CT angiography may be performed. As an alternative, ultrasound imaging of the IVC inferior vena cava and right ventricular (RV) volume overload may be utilized at the bedside. The addition of AI artificial intelligence automated cardiac imaging analysis (recently cleared by the FDA and European CE mark authorities) is important since the RV is difficult to evaluate due to its unique structure and location. Regarding Covid-19 mortality, recent studies show a significant link between right heart failure and an Mt. Sinai Med Center study showed 31% of patients hospitalized with COVID-19 had right ventricle failure and 41% of this subset who died had findings of right ventricular dilation or enlargement. Cardiomyopathy may be incidentally found and further studied with other radiographic and imaging technologies.

2.4   Image Guided Fusion Treatments

Concerns over increasing use of CT and increasing radiation burden have prompted efforts to reduce associated radiation dose especially in the pediatric population. With the reduction in radiation dose, if scan and reconstruction factors are held constant, the image quality decreases, however, such dose reduction and loss of image quality may not compromise the diagnostic evaluation of some anatomic regions and evaluation. However, for other body regions and abnormalities, decreased image quality at lower radiation dose can reduce the diagnostic information. To maintain or improve CT image quality at low radiation dose, vendors developed improved scanner hardware (such as better detector efficiency) and iterative reconstruction (IR) techniques. Traditional filtered back-projection (FBP) reconstruction methods enable fast computation of CT data but are prone to increased noise and artifacts at low radiation doses. The addition of FUSION imaging with high resolution LUS may enhance the role of millisevert CT as benefits image guided treatment options, such as fluid sampling and image-guided interventions. Cross-sectional image guided interventional procedures are performed under CT, ultrasound, fluoroscopy, or MRI guidance and include fluid aspiration, (thoracentesis, paracentesis, and fluid collections), drainage catheter placement, percutaneous biopsy, and tumor ablation. It is useful to pre-procedure map the vascular and possible neural structures pertinent to the treatment field with Doppler ultrasound to avoid unnecessary blood loss, nerve damage, and accidental perforation of significant vessels.

2.4.1   Bedside Lung and IVC Imaging

In the 10 months since COVID-19 became a worldwide epidemic, lung ultrasound now accompanies most patients as a precursor or postcursor imaging modality. In critical cases where pulmonary emboli is suspected, CT angiography may be performed. As an alternative, ultrasound imaging of the IVC inferior vena cava and right ventricular (RV) volume overload may be utilized at the bedside. The addition of AI artificial intelligence automated cardiac imaging analysis (recently cleared by the FDA and European CE mark authorities) is important since the RV is difficult to evaluate due to its unique structure and location. Regarding COVID-19 mortality, recent studies show a significant link between right heart failure and a Mt. Sinai Medical Center (New York City) study showed 31% of patients hospitalized with COVID-19 had right ventricle failure and 41% of this subset who died had findings of right ventricular dilation or enlargement. Since bedside diagnostics are currently normalized worldwide, it is useful to differentiate acute pulmonary disease from acute heart failure (AHF) during the routine lung ultrasound exploration. Point of care ultrasound (POCUS) of the inferior vena cava (IVC) is accepted as a quick and useful modality for diagnosis and determination of prognosis of patients with AHF. A study of the IVC using IVC expiratory diameter and/or IVC collapsibility index demonstrated an IVC expiratory dimension greater than 2.0 cm and an IVC collapsibility index of less than 30% suggest that acute dyspnea is likely to be due to AHF [20].

2.5   Image Guided Procedures

CT, CT-LUS fusion and sonography-guided punctures have a low rate of complications. The rate of pneumothorax is 2.8%; 1% require drainage. Hemorrhage or hemoptysis is observed in 0–2%. Data concerning air embolism or even death are not available so far. Tumor dissemination through the procedure of puncture is of little clinical significance and very rare, in less than 0.003% of cases. In cases of malignant pleural mesothelioma, it is slightly more common. When surgery is performed, the site of puncture is also resected.

2.5.1   Pneumothorax After Puncture

If the focus of the procedure is no longer visible after the puncture, the likelihood of a pneumothorax is high. This can be reliably detected by sonography, through the absence of respiration-dependent gliding movement of the pleura. The quantity of free air can only be measured by obtaining a chest radiograph or limited CT scan. A pneumothorax usually reaches its maximum dimensions after 3 h, so the decision regarding a therapeutic procedure is made thereafter, when the pneumothorax is smaller. If the patient is symptomatic or if a larger volume is present, the patient is initially given protracted thoracocentesis. The success rate within the first 10 h is 90%. In the event of renewed collapse, the clinician may use a percutaneous drain and a catheter with a small lumen. A routine chest radiograph or follow up CT scan is not required after routine CT or sonography-guided puncture.

Prognosis is related to the chest wall pleural thickness, which is better demonstrated on sequential high resolution sonography and not as clinically practical in CT imaging in recovering patients.

2.6   Radiographic Limitations

Since most cases will need to be correlated with X-ray or CT findings, it is important to note the limitations of X-ray and CT findings. X-ray misses most early Covid disease but is useful in finding the more advanced pneumonic consolidation process. It is impossible to differentiate COVID-19 typical image findings from other diseases. For example, bacterial pneumonia can present with focal segmental or lobar pulmonary opacities without lower lung predominance, but other common findings (cavitation, lung abscess, lymphadenopathy, and so on) can usually differentiate it from COVID-19. Other viral pneumonias are more challenging to distinguish from COVID-19. For example, ground-glass opacities (GGOs) can be seen in up to 75% of adenovirus cases, more than 75% of cytomegalovirus and herpes simplex virus cases, and up to 25% of measles and human meta-pneumovirus cases. GGOs can be widespread in pneumocystis pneumonia, but, unlike in COVID-19, they tend to predominate in the upper lobes. Similarly, various interstitial lung diseases can present with GGOs, but the predominant location differs by diagnosis, and other clinical factors are useful for differentiating them from COVID-19.

GGOs can also be common in hypersensitivity pneumonitis, lung injury from use of electronic cigarettes or vaping products, pulmonary edema, diffuse alveolar hemorrhage, pulmonary alveolar proteinosis, and eosinophilic pneumonia. But clinical features and GGO patterns are generally useful for differentiating these conditions from COVID-19. CT is valuable in identifying underlying cardiopulmonary abnormalities in patients with moderate to severe disease. CT can help clinicians triage resources toward patients at risk of disease progression and may identify a cause in case of clinical worsening. CT may also identify alternate diagnoses. Dr. Marcello Migliore of the University of Catania, in Italy, who recently reviewed the management of GGOs in the lung cancer screening era, told Reuters Health by email, "CT is not useful to diagnose COVID-19, but it is certainly useful to follow up patients with preexisting lung pathology who go rapidly worse. However, GGOs are also a presenting picture of early lung cancer and therefore it should be taken into account." Another use is to follow patients with mild GGO initial CT findings since a certain percentage develop pleural fibrosis and increasing respiratory compromise even as the opacities clear.

References

1. World Health Organization website. Emergencies preparedness, response: novel coronavirus—China. 2020. www.who.int/csr/don/12-january-2020-novel-coronavirus-china/en/. Accessed 14 Apr 2020.
2. World Health Organization website. WHO director-general's remarks at the media briefing on 2019-nCoV on 11 February 2020. 2020. www.who.int/dg/speeches/detail/who-director-general-s-remarks-at-the-media-briefing-on-2019-ncov-on-11-february-2020. Accessed 14 Apr 2020.
3. International Committee on Taxonomy of Viruses website. Naming the 2019 coronavirus. 2020. talk.ictvonline.org/. Accessed 14 Apr 2020.
4. World Health Organization website. Emergencies preparedness, response: pneumonia of unknown cause in China. 2020. www.who.int/csr/don/05-january-2020-pneumonia-of-unkown-cause-china/en/. Accessed 14 Apr 2020.
5. China National Health Commission website. Diagnosis and treatment of pneumonitis caused by new coronavirus (trial version 5). 2020. www.nhc.gov.cn/yzygj/s7653p/202002/3b09b894ac9b4204a79db5b8912d4440.shtml. Accessed 14 Apr 2020.
6. China National Health Commission website. Diagnosis and treatment of pneumonitis caused by new coronavirus (trial version 5, revision). 2020. www.nhc.gov.cn/yzygj/s7653p/202002/d4b895337e19445f8d728fcaf1e3e13a.shtml. Accessed 14 Apr 2020.
7. Huang P, Liu T, Huang L, et al. Use of chest CT in combination with negative RT-PCR assay for the 2019 novel coronavirus but high clinical suspicion. Radiology. 2020;295:22–3.

8. Ai T, Yang Z, Hou H, et al. Correlation of chest CT and RT-PCR testing in coronavirus disease 2019 (COVID-19) in China: a report of 1014 cases. Radiology. 2020;296(2):E32–40.
9. Chung M, Bernheim A, Mei X, et al. CT imaging features of 2019 novel coronavirus (2019-nCoV). Radiology. 2020;295:202–7.
10. Han R, Huang L, Jiang H, Dong J, Peng H, Zhang D. Early clinical and CT manifestations of coronavirus disease 2019 (COVID-19) pneumonia. AJR. 2020;215(2):338–43.
11. Huang C, Wang Y, Li X, et al. Clinical features of patients infected with 2019 novel coronavirus in Wuhan, China. Lancet. 2020;395:497–506.
12. Li M, Lei P, Zeng B, et al. Coronavirus disease (COVID-19): spectrum of CT findings and temporal progression of the disease. Acad Radiol. 2020;27(5):603–8.
13. Song F, Shi N, Shan F, et al. Emerging 2019 novel coronavirus (2019-nCoV) pneumonia. Radiology. 2020;295:210–7.
14. Chan JF, Yuan S, Kok KH, et al. A familial cluster of pneumonia associated with the 2019 novel coronavirus indicating person-to-person transmission: a study of a family cluster. Lancet. 2020;395:514–23.
15. Kanne JP. Chest CT findings in 2019 novel coronavirus (2019-nCoV) infections from Wuhan, China: key points for the radiologist. Radiology. 2020;295:16–7.
16. Xie X, Zhong Z, Zhao W, Zheng C, Wang F, Liu J. Chest CT for typical 2019-nCoV pneumonia: relationship to negative RT-PCR testing. Radiology. 2020;296(2):E41–5.
17. Kim EA, Lee KS, Primack SL, et al. Viral pneumonias in adults: radiopathologic findings. Radiographics. 2002;22:137–49.
18. Lin L, Gangze F, Chen S, et al. CT manifestations of Covid-19 pneumonia and influenza virus pneumonia. AJR. 2020;215:1–9.
19. Han R, Huang L, Jiang H, et al. Can chest CT distinguish patients with negative from those with positive initial RT-PCR results for Covid-19. AJR. 2020;215:106–18.
20. Darwish O, Mahani A, Kataria S, et al. Diagnosis of acute heart failure using inferior vena cava ultrasound. J Ultrasound Med. 2020;39:1367–78.

Lung Ultrasound in COVID-19 Disease

3

Dirk-André Clevert and Felix Escher

3.1   Introduction

Due to the rapid increase in SARS-CoV-2 (COVID-19) cases worldwide, the World Health Organization has announced a pandemic [1].

In most of the cases, COVID-19 causes mild symptoms such as fever (80%), dry cough (56%), fatigue (22%) and limb pain (7%) [2]. However, severe courses of the disease are associated with pneumonia and respiratory failure requiring intensive care support [2, 3]. Elderly patients and those with comorbidities such as immune disorders or cardiovascular diseases have a higher risk in developing an acute respiratory distress syndrome (ARDS) as well as further life-threatening complications including septic shock [2]. The wide and simultaneous spread of the infection with the need for advanced health care support makes this pandemic a real health emergency [4].

Critically ill patients frequently need thoracic imaging due to the constant changes of their clinical conditions [5]. A key part of monitoring critical patients in the intensive care unit (ICU) and emergency room (ER) is thoracic ultrasound as it allows a thorough examination of both the lung and pleural space [6]. Patients with COVID-19 disease show typically patterns in computed tomography (CT) scans like diffuse bilateral interstitial pneumonia, with asymmetric, patchy lesions distributed mainly in the periphery of the lung [7–9].

Supplementary Information The online version of this chapter (https://doi.org/10.1007/978-3-030-66614-9_3) contains supplementary material, which is available to authorized users.

D.-A. Clevert (✉) · F. Escher
Interdisciplinary Ultrasound-Center, Department of Radiology, University of Munich-Grosshadern Campus, Munich, Germany
e-mail: dirk.clevert@med.uni-muenchen.de; felix.escher@med.uni-muenchen.de

Chest CT is still regarded as the gold standard imaging technique for thoracic evaluation. Nevertheless, it has important disadvantages as transportation of patients outside the Intensive Care Unit (ICU) is difficult and potentially harmful [10]. Furthermore, CT scans expose patients to radiation and should be reserved for specific situations (e.g., the evaluation of mediastinal pathologies and confirmation of pulmonary embolism) [11–13]. Bedside chest X-ray (CXR) is still considered standard of care for many diagnostic applications in the ICU and emergency room (ER). However, this imaging technique has important methodological limitations and often shows low accuracy [14]. As lung abnormalities may develop before clinical manifestations and nucleic acid detection, experts have recommended early chest computerized tomography (CT) for screening suspected patients [15]. The high contagiousness of COVID-19 and the risk of transport of unstable patients with hypoxemia and hemodynamic failure make chest CTs a limited option for the patient with suspected or established COVID-19 [10].

With regards to the evaluation of pneumonia and/or ARDS lung ultrasonography (LUS) provides results comparable to chest CT and superior to standard CXR with the added advantage of ease of use at point of care, repeatability, absence of radiation exposure, and low cost [15, 16]. The use of this ultrasound technique could reduce both CXR and CT in ICUs and ERs [6].

3.2   Basics of Lung Ultrasound Examinations

Thorax and lung ultrasound have gained importance in daily clinical routine [17–22] which is especially true in the setting of point of care ultrasound (POCUS) [23] (Figs. 3.1 and 3.2).

The first sonographic examinations of the lung were performed more than 50 years ago [24, 25] although the lung was not considered suitable for this imaging technology at first [26–28].

Acute dyspnoea is a common leading symptom in the ER and on the ICU and the range of possible differential diagnoses is broad. After careful anamnesis, physical examination and checking vital signs a prompt POCUS should be performed.

Fig. 3.1 Dynamic examination of the intercostal muscles. Enlargement of the muscle during expiration

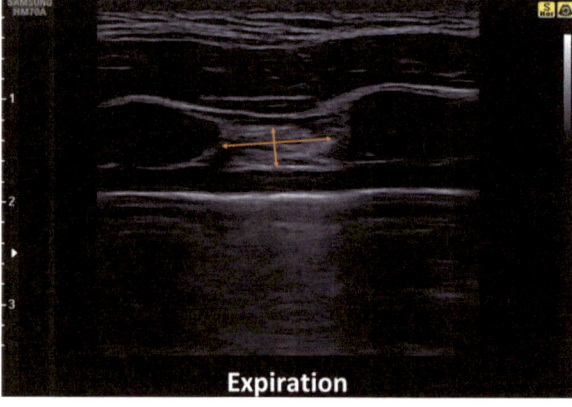

Fig. 3.2 Dynamic examination of the intercostal muscles. Contraction of the muscle during inspiration

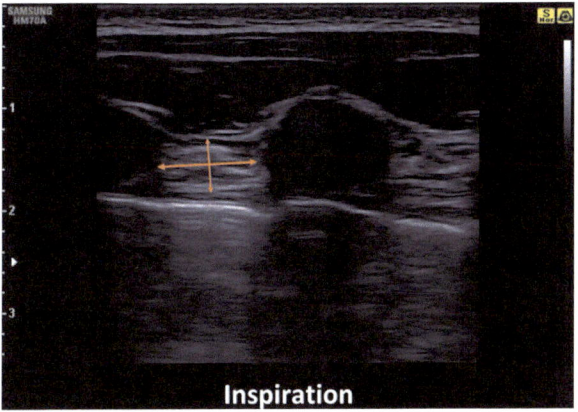

Alongside echocardiography and abdominal sonography, LUS plays a crucial role in the field of emergency sonography. Despite existing recommendations for elective chest sonography [29, 30] and emergency pulmonary sonography [17], point of care pulmonary sonography has not yet been widely established in daily practice [31]. Compared to clinical examination and chest X-ray, pulmonary sonography shows excellent diagnostic accuracy in diagnosing pleural effusions, pneumothorax, pulmonary venous congestion and consolidation [14, 32, 33]. In order to diagnose lung pathologies, we use ultrasound artifacts that occur due to different characteristics of the chest wall and pleural surface. These artifacts contain valuable information and correlate with the current lung pathophysiology. The two predominant artifact patterns are "A-lines" and "B-lines" [34].

3.2.1   A-lines

A-lines are reverberation artifacts caused by oscillating. Due to differences in acoustic impedance between tissue and air ultrasound waves are reflected strongly and bounce back and forth between the transducer and lung surface [15, 35]. A-lines are defined as parallel horizontal repetition lines of the pleura in the depth. As A-lines are classic reverberation artifacts, the distance from the skin to the pleural line equals the distance from the pleural line to the first A-line and equals the distance from the first A-line to the second A-line, and so forth (Fig. 3.3).

The so-called A profile is formed by an intact ("dry") lung parenchyma containing air and simultaneous presence of physiological lung sliding. Absence of lung sliding is highly suggestive of pneumothorax [36].

3.2.2   B-lines

The "comet-tail" ultrasonographic sign was first described by Ziskin and colleagues in 1982 when an intrahepatic shotgun pellet was observed to create an artifact

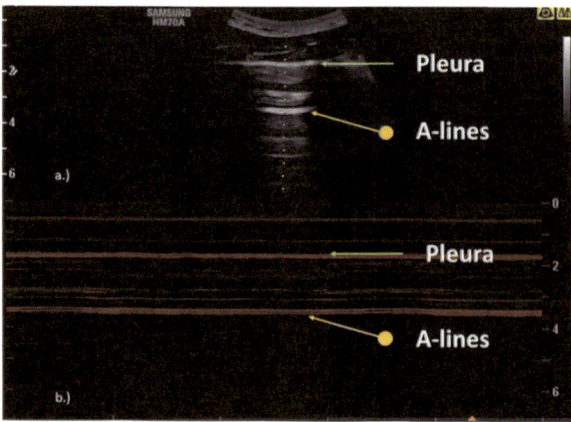

Fig. 3.3 Ultrasound image demonstrating A-lines by using a curve array probe. The A-lines are clearly visible on the M-mode and B-mode as bright white lines (yellow arrows). The A-lines are the bright horizontal lines deep to the pleural line (green arrows). A-lines are a classic reverberation artifact. The distance from the skin to the pleural line equals the distance from the pleural line to the first A-line

Fig. 3.4 Ultrasound image demonstrating comet-tail artifacts (yellow arrows), the artifact originates at the pleura (green arrow) but fades

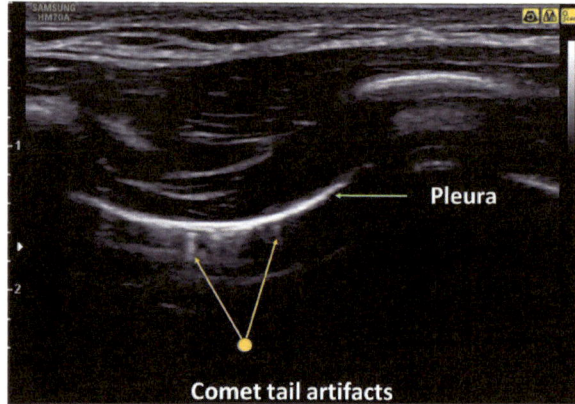

similar to what is seen in lung comets [36] (Fig. 3.4). B-lines should not be confused with normal comet-tail artifacts that originate at the pleura but fade before reaching the edge of the screen.

B-lines are vertical, highly dynamic, hyperechoic artifacts originating from the pleura or consolidation areas [37]. These lines indicate accumulation of fluid in the pulmonary interstitial space ("lung rockets") or alveoli ("ground glass"). Multiple B-lines are associated with pulmonary edema of cardiogenic (mostly anterior ground glass), noncardiogenic (ARDS), or mixed origin (Fig. 3.5). They occur when sound waves pass through superficial soft tissues and cross the pleural line encountering a mixture of air and water. As a rule of thumb, one or two B-lines are not too concerning but when they increase in number or spread out in one zone, they are a sign of a present interstitial pathology (Fig. 3.6).

3.3   Transducer Selection and Settings

Conventional ultrasound systems with a "real-time B-mode" technique are suitable for preoperative and postoperative transthoracic ultrasound. Several ultrasonography probes are eligible for LUS with each having specific advantages and limitations. The choice depends on multiple factors such as anatomy, size and age of the patient, depth and nature of the structures to be visualized and the specific goals of the investigation. In recent years, however, prospective studies using high-frequency linear, low-frequency curvilinear and low-frequency sector transducers have demonstrated that both performance and interpretation of LUS are not transducer-specific [38]. Keep in mind that low-frequency transducers will provide more depth penetration but sacrifice image quality; in turn, high-frequency transducers will show better resolution but sacrifice depth penetration [36].

3.3.1   Convex Transducers

Low-frequency convex transducers are more suitable for bedside lung ultrasonography because they can be used to visualize the deep posterior-lateral structures and can reveal consolidations and pleural effusion [35] (Fig. 3.7).

3.3.2   Linear Transducers

However, low-penetration, high-frequency, and high-definition linear transducers may be preferable for identifying pneumothorax and examining the superficial

Fig. 3.5 Examination of the lung using a linear array probe. B-lines (yellow arrows) are vertical hyperechoic reverberation artifacts that arise from the pleural line (green arrow), extend to the bottom of the screen without fading

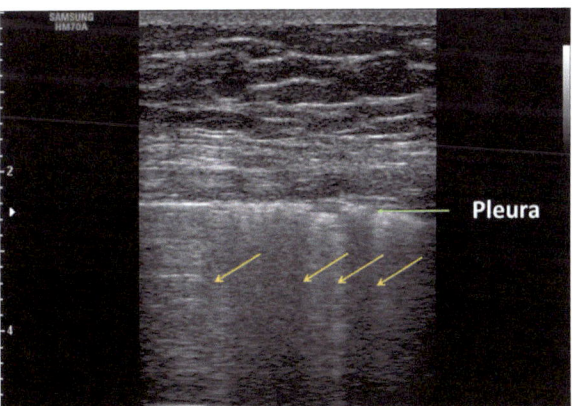

Fig. 3.6 One or two B-lines (yellow arrows) are not too concerning but when they increase in number or spread out in one zone, they are a sign of a present interstitial pathology

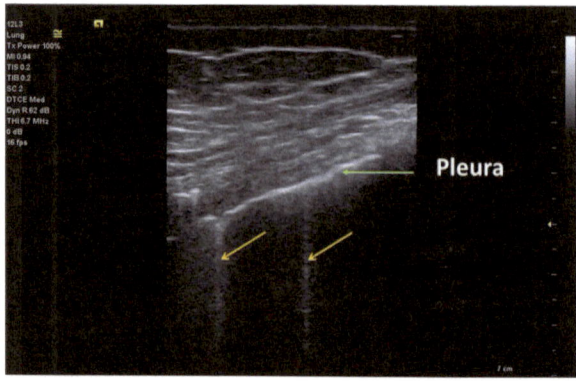

Fig. 3.7 Ultrasound image demonstrating A-lines by using a curve array probe. The A-lines (yellow arrows) are the bright horizontal lines deep to the pleural line (green arrow)

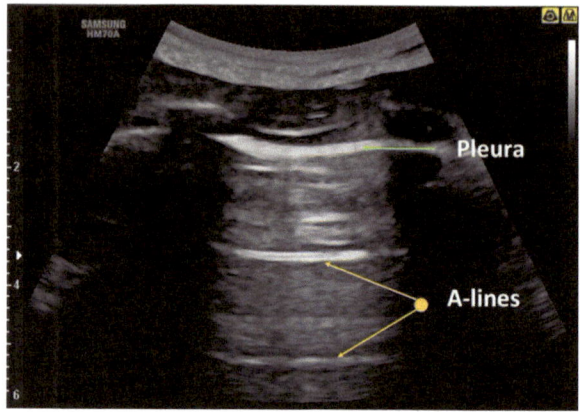

anterior structures (i.e., pleural line lung sliding) in both children and thin adults (Fig. 3.8).

3.3.3 Phased and Microconvex Transducers

Phased and microconvex transducers are used for a wide range of indications including consolidation and pleural effusion. Basic ultrasound units should be equipped with pulsed and color Doppler as well as M-mode in order to be able to evaluate vessels and the vascularization of pathologies [39]. In addition to the standard B-mode, the diagnostic value of ultrasound can be improved by using the dynamic M-mode. By using the M-mode, a single vertical line of the ultrasound image is selected. The ultrasound signals of this line are displayed over time in a separate diagram allowing movements in the tissue to be represented as curves. Immobile structures appear as horizontal lines. When M-mode is applied to the lung exam, the system displays a representation of tissue motion over time [35].

Fig. 3.8 Ultrasound image demonstrating A-lines (yellow arrows) by using a linear probe. The A-lines are the bright horizontal lines deep to the pleural line (green arrow)

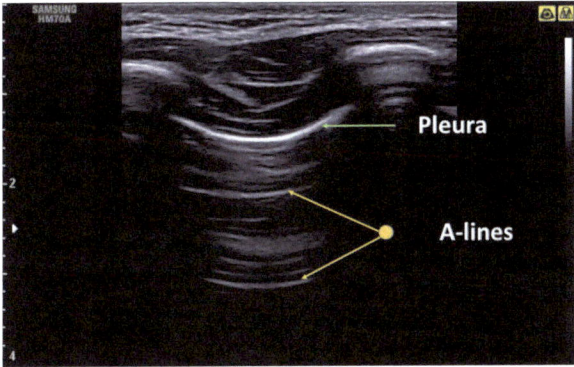

Most ultrasound manufacturers use further technical processes for image enhancement, such as compound imaging and harmonic imaging resulting in overall better image quality necessary for a conventional examination. However, disabling these modes will result in a clearer display of comet-tail artifacts or B-lines [35]. Adjustments to focal zone, image depth and overall gain should be made for optimal visualization of the pleural line [40].

3.4   Examination Procedure and Pathologies

LUS is used in emergency and intensive care patients in lying (ventral thorax) and—depending on the clinical setting—in a sitting position (dorsal thorax). A systematic approach investigating the entire anterolateral and posterior lung surfaces bilaterally should be used. In some cases, a patient-focused abbreviated approach may be useful.

Each hemithorax should be divided into six regions [41]. Anterior and posterior axillary lines serve as landmarks to divide each hemithorax into anterior, lateral, and posterior regions; then an axial line will serve to divide the upper and lower regions [42]. The six regions for each hemithorax, anterior superior, anterior inferior, lateral superior, lateral inferior, posterior superior, and posterior inferior, should be marked as R1–R6 and L1–L6, respectively.

Typically, the transthoracic scanning window will be used for the examination of the lung and pleura [31]. The intercostal spaces serve as additional scanning windows. The convex array transducer should be positioned rectangular to the ribs so that two adjacent ribs are captured. This allows reliable identification of lung sliding, i.e., the movement of the pleura visceralis. By using this technique each intercostal space of upper and lower parts of the anterior, lateral, and posterior regions of the left and right chest wall are carefully examined [43]. Finally, a linear array transducer may be helpful in evaluating suspected subpleural lesions.

3.5   Image Fusion

For complex lung pathologies, real-time ultrasound image fusion with high-resolution CT (HR-CT) datasets can be performed using high-end ultrasound systems. This is especially useful for severely ill patients in the ICU, as this technique allows pathologies to be monitored directly at the bedside. This could lead to a further reduction of CT examinations and minimizes the risk of contamination due to less patient transports.

Ultrasound fusion requires additional hardware such as a magnetic field generator and position sensors. The position sensor is used to localize the position of the transducer in the three-dimensional space. Image fusion is possible with most imaging modalities including CT. DICOM (digital imaging and communication in medicine) datasets of HR-CT scans can be coregistered with the help of the ultrasound system software and can be viewed in a side-by-side mode or in an overlay mode in real-time [44].

During image fusion, other image modes of the ultrasound system such as color Doppler and CEUS may still be used. Using multiple image techniques in real-time allows comprehensive imaging and characterization of the vascularization of lung pathologies [45]. Fusion imaging could help in the detection and localization of lung lesions with low conspicuity on standard B-mode ultrasound. In abdominal imaging and animal studies, image fusion is already being used on several organs [44, 46–55].

3.6   Findings

Compared to non-COVID-19 pneumonia, COVID-19 pneumonia is more likely to show a peripheral distribution making it accessible for ultrasound evaluation as lesions are localized close to the pleura [56]. In addition to HR-CT, ultrasound can also be used for both diagnosis and follow-up of COVID-19 [14].

By using a curved transducer, the morphology, and changes of subpleural lesions are clearly displayed. With low-frequency transducers, changes of air and water contents in consolidated peri-pulmonary tissues and air bronchogram signs can be depicted.

Currently, LUS is limited in the diagnosis and treatment of central lung diseases due to the attenuation of sound waves by normal lung and bone tissues. Therefore, diagnosis of lung pathologies relies on artifacts of peri-pulmonary lesions [57, 58].

The artifacts exist due to the abnormal ratio of air and water contents in alveoli and interstitial tissues. In order to improve the diagnostic ultrasound lung tool, the use of an abdominal curved array probe seems to be helpful in our study (Figs. 3.9, 3.10, and 3.11). Typical for the COVID-19 disease are the thickening of the pleural line with pleural line irregularity. The pleural line's appearance may be either unsmooth, discontinuous or interrupted [14, 59].

The appearance of B-lines artifacts (<3 B-lines per intercostal space) varies from focal, multifocal to confluent patterns [16]. Consolidations show different patterns including multifocal small subpleural consolidations up to non-translobar and translobar patterns with occasional air bronchograms [60].

Fig. 3.9 Examination of the lung using curved array probe. In comparison to Fig. 3.6, increase in the B-lines (yellow arrows). The pleural line appears partially interrupted (green arrow)

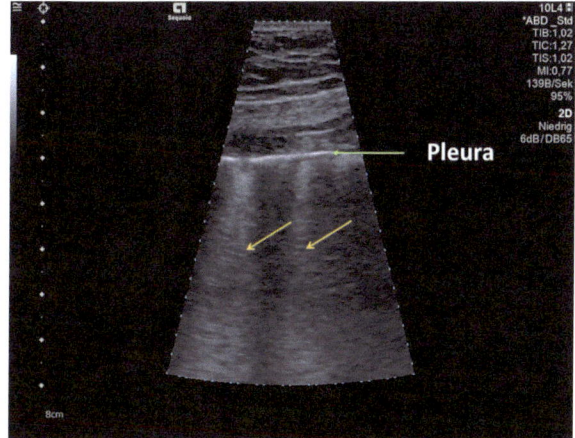

Fig. 3.10 Examination of the lung using a curved array transducer. Fragmentation of the pleura (yellow arrows) with consolidations

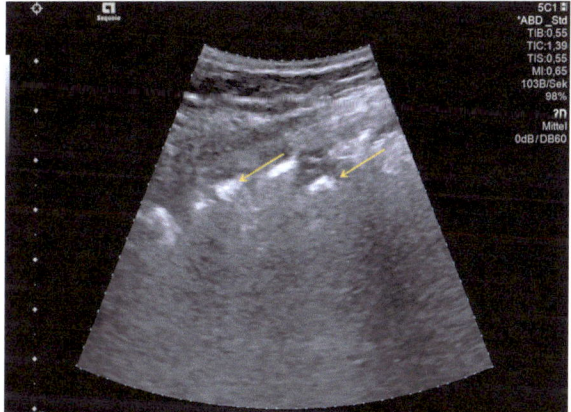

Fig. 3.11 Examination of the lung using a curved array transducer. Pleura effusion (white arrow) and multiple B-lines (yellow arrows). Additionally fragmentation of the pleura is visible (green arrow)

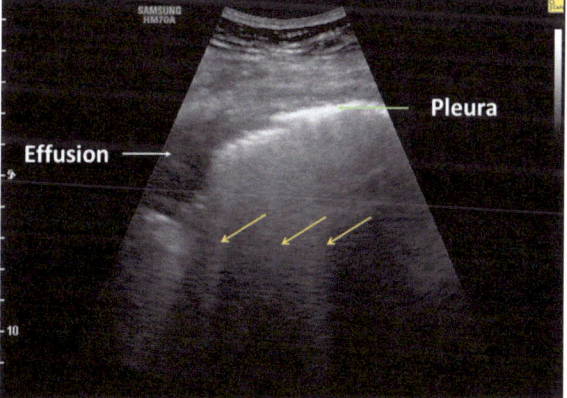

Pleural effusions are uncommon in COVID-19 disease. In our experience, pleural effusions seem to be associated with more severe courses of the disease. The appearance of A-lines during the recovery phase may be interpreted as an indirect sign for recovering [15].

In summary, in our experience, we consider that LUS will have a major benefit for the management of COVID-19 pneumonia in the ICU and ER due to its safety, repeatability, low cost and point of care use [61]. HR-CT should be reserved in the follow-up if LUS is not able to answer the clinical question. In our personal experience LUS could be used for rapid severity assessment of COVID-19 pneumonia, to track the course of the disease during follow-up and to monitor lung recruitment maneuvers. Moreover, ultrasound can track the patient's response to prone position and is helpful in the management of extracorporeal membrane therapy [15]. With increased use of bedside ultrasound in the ICU and ER, patients can be protected from unnecessary radiation and therapy delays [62]. In addition, transport of high-risk patients to CT examinations can be avoided. The use of image fusion makes it possible to fuse CT and ultrasound images in real time in order to detect a possible progression of the disease in comparison to the last CT (Figs. 3.12 and 3.13).

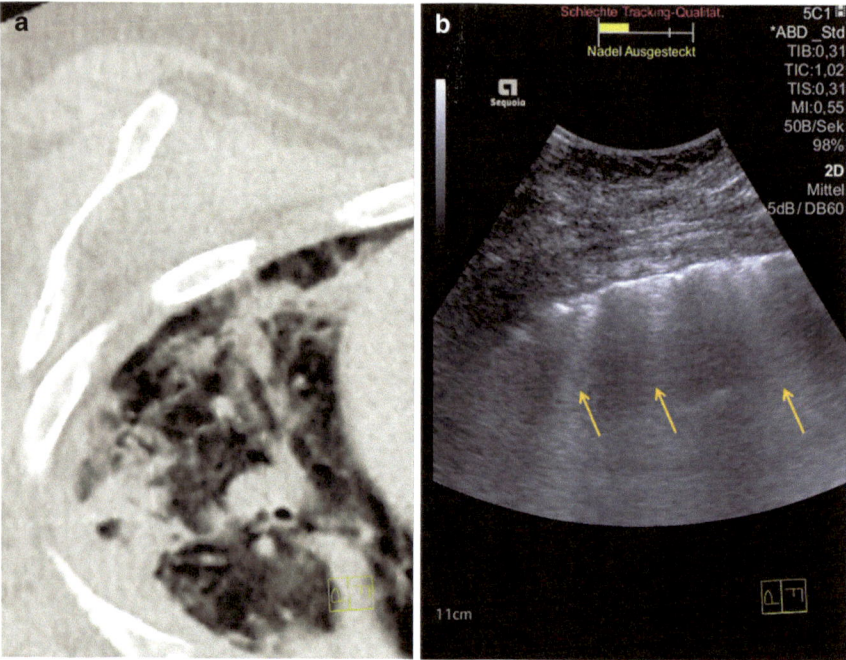

Fig. 3.12 Image fusion examination of the lung with simultaneous acquisition of CT data (**a**) and ultrasound data (**b**) in real time. Both modalities show consolidation in the CT and ultrasound image (yellow arrows)

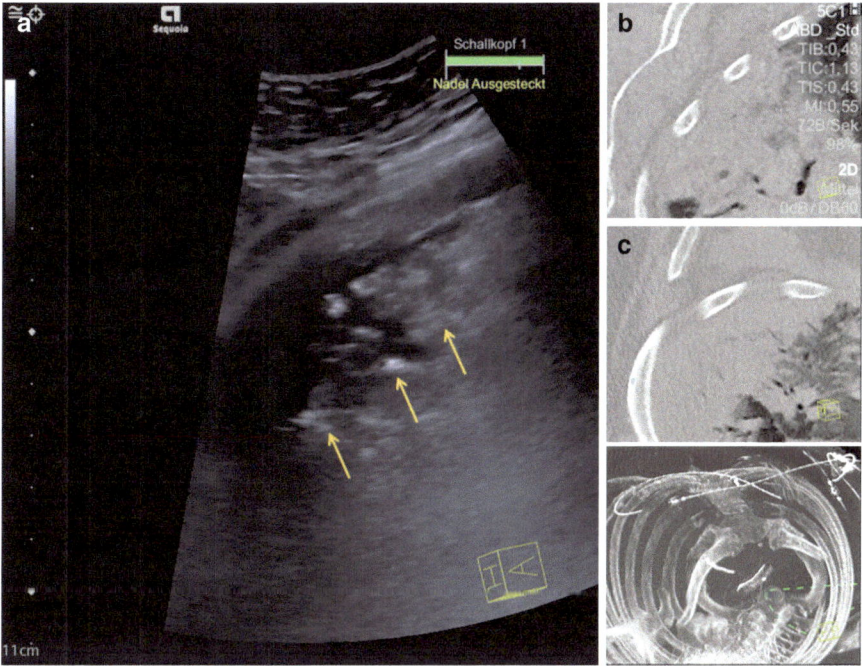

Fig. 3.13 Follow-up examination on the ICU by using the real-time image fusion technic with a curved array probe. HR-CT (**b, c**) showed large flaps of soft tissues and low-density shadows under the pleura additionally ultrasound (**a**) detected large air bronchogram sign (yellow arrows) in the image fusion technic

3.7   Conclusions

In summary, patients with COVID-19 disease show typical patterns in lung ultrasound. COVID-19 lesions mainly involve the peripheral pulmonary zones which makes this disease accessible for pulmonary ultrasound evaluation [42]. We consider that LUS offers major benefits in managing COVID-19 pneumonia in both the ICU and ER due to its noninvasive assessment and dynamic observation of lung lesions. The major advantages of LUS are the safety, the repeatability as well as the low cost in point of care. With increased use of bedside ultrasound, patients can be protected from unnecessary radiation and therapy delays. The number of transports of high-risk patients to CT examinations could be reduced. Image fusion is a helpful tool in monitoring selected cases on the ICU.

References

1. Cucinotta D, Vanelli M. WHO declares COVID-19 a pandemic. Acta Biomed. 2020;91(1):157–60. https://doi.org/10.23750/abm.v91i1.9397.
2. Wujtewicz M, Dylczyk-Sommer A, Aszkiełowicz A, Zdanowski S, Piwowarczyk S, Owczuk R. COVID-19 - what should anaethesiologists and intensivists know about it? Anaesthesiol Intensive Ther. 2020; https://doi.org/10.5114/ait.2020.93756.
3. Zhu N, Zhang D, Wang W, Li X, et al. A novel coronavirus from patients with pneumonia in China. N Engl J Med. 2020;382:727–33. https://doi.org/10.1056/NEJMoa2001017.
4. Soldati G, Giannasi G, Smargiassi A, Inchingolo R, Demi L. Contrast-enhanced ultrasound in patients with COVID-19: pneumonia, acute respiratory distress syndrome, or something else? J Ultrasound Med. 2020; https://doi.org/10.1002/jum.15338.
5. Brogi E, Bignami E, Sidoti A, Shawar M, Gargani L, Vetrugno L, Volpicelli G, Forfori F. Could the use of bedside lung ultrasound reduce the number of chest x-rays in the intensive care unit? Cardiovasc Ultrasound. 2017;15(1):23. https://doi.org/10.1186/s12947-017-0113-8.
6. Oks M, Cleven KL, Cardenas-Garcia J, Schaub JA, Koenig S, Cohen RI, Mayo PH, Narasimhan M. The effect of point-of-care ultrasonography on imaging studies in the medical ICU: a comparative study. Chest. 2014;146:1574–7. https://doi.org/10.1378/chest.14-0728.
7. Wu J, Wu X, Zeng W, et al. Chest CT findings in patients with corona virus disease 2019 and its relationship with clinical features. Investig Radiol. 2020;55(5):257–61. https://doi.org/10.1097/RLI.0000000000000670.
8. Zhao W, Zhong Z, Xie X, Yu Q, Liu J. Relation between chest CT findings and clinical conditions of coronavirus disease (COVID-19) pneumonia: a multicenter study. AJR Am J Roentgenol. 2020;214(5):1072–7. https://doi.org/10.2214/AJR.20.22976.
9. Zhou S, Wang Y, Zhu T, Xia L. T features of coronavirus disease 2019 (COVID-19) pneumonia in 62 patients in Wuhan, China. AJR Am J Roentgenol China. 2020;214(6):1287–94. https://doi.org/10.2214/AJR.20.22975.
10. Dunn MJ, Gwinnutt CL, Gray AJ. Critical care in the emergency department: patient transfer. Emerg Med J. 2007;24(1):40–4. https://doi.org/10.1136/emj.2006.042044.
11. Tecce PM, Fishman EK, Kuhlman JE. CT evaluation of the anterior mediastinum: spectrum of disease. Radiographics. 1994;14(5):973–90. https://doi.org/10.1148/radiographics.14.5.7991827.
12. Brenner DJ, Hall EJ. Computed tomography–an increasing source of radiation exposure. N Engl J Med. 2007;357(22):2277–84. https://doi.org/10.1056/NEJMra072149.
13. Tapson VF. Advances in the diagnosis and treatment of acute pulmonary embolism. F1000 Med Rep. 2012;4:9. https://doi.org/10.3410/M4-9.
14. Lichtenstein D, Goldstein I, Mourgeon E, Cluzel P, Grenier P, Rouby JJ. Comparative diagnostic performances of auscultation, chest radiography, and lung ultrasonography in acute respiratory distress syndrome. Anesthesiology. 2004;100(1):9–15. https://doi.org/10.1097/00000542-200401000-00006.
15. Peng QY, Wang XT, Zhang LN, Chinese Critical Care Ultrasound Study Group (CCUSG). Findings of lung ultrasonography of novel corona virus pneumonia during the 2019-2020 epidemic. Intensive Care Med. 2020;46:849–50. https://doi.org/10.1007/s00134-020-05996-6.
16. Mayo PH, Copetti R, Feller-Kopman D, Mathis G, Maury E, Mongodi S, Mojoli F, Volpicelli G, Zanobetti M. Thoracic ultrasonography: a narrative review. Intensive Care Med. 2019;45:1200–11. https://doi.org/10.1007/s00134-019-05725-8.
17. Volpicelli G, Elbarbary M, Blaivas M, et al. International evidence-based recommendations for point-of-care lung ultrasound. Intensive Care Med. 2012;38:577–91. https://doi.org/10.1007/s00134-012-2513-4.
18. Volpicelli G. Lung sonography. J Ultrasound Med. 2013;32:165–71. https://doi.org/10.7863/jum.2013.32.1.165.
19. Dietrich CF, Gebhard Mathis G, Cui XW, et al. Ultrasound of the pleurae and lungs. Ultrasound Med Biol. 2015;41:351–65. https://doi.org/10.1016/j.ultrasmedbio.2014.10.002.

20. Mathis G. Why look for artifacts alone when the original is visible? Chest. 2010;137:233.; author reply 233–4. https://doi.org/10.1378/chest.08-2601.
21. Gargani L, Pang PS, Frassi F, et al. Persistent pulmonary congestion before discharge predicts rehospitalization in heart failure: a lung ultrasound study. Cardiovasc Ultrasound. 2015;13:40. https://doi.org/10.1186/s12947-015-0033-4.
22. Gargani L. Lung ultrasound: a new tool for the cardiologist. Cardiovasc Ultrasound. 2011;9:6. https://doi.org/10.1186/1476-7120-9-6.
23. Bouhemad B, Liu ZH, Arbelot C, et al. Ultrasound assessment of antibiotic-induced pulmonary reaeration in ventilator-associated pneumonia. Crit Care Med. 2010;38:84–92. https://doi.org/10.1097/CCM.0b013e3181b08cdb.
24. Buddee FW, Johnson DC, Jellins J. Experimental and clinical experiences in the use of ultrasound for the early detection of pulmonary emboli: a preliminary report. Med J Aust. 1969;1:295–7. https://doi.org/10.5694/j.1326-5377.1969.tb92130.x.
25. Crawford HD, Wild JJ, Wolf PI, Finks JS. Transmission of ultrasound through living human thorax. IRE Trans Med Electron. 1959:141–6.
26. Lichtenstein DA. BLUE-protocol and FALLS-protocol: two applications of lung ultrasound in the critically ill. Chest. 2015;147(6):1659–70. https://doi.org/10.1378/chest.14-1313.
27. Weinberger SE, Drazen JM. Diagnostic procedures in respiratory diseases. In: Kasper DL, Braunwald E, Fauci AS, Hauser SL, Longo DL, Jameson JL, editors. harrison's principles of internal medicine. 16th ed. New York, NY: McGraw-Hill; 2005. p. 1505–8.
28. Mayo PH, Beaulieu Y, Doelken P, et al. American College of Chest Physicians/La Société de Réanimation de Langue Française statement on competence in critical care ultrasonography. Chest. 2009;135(4):1050–60. https://doi.org/10.1378/chest.08-2305.
29. Havelock T, Teoh R, Laws D, et al. Pleural procedures and thoracic ultrasound: British Thoracic Society pleural disease guideline 2010. Thorax. 2010;65(Suppl 2):61–76.
30. Piscaglia F, Nolsoe C, Dietrich CF, et al. The EFSUMB guidelines and recommendations on the clinical practice of contrast enhanced ultrasound (CEUS): update 2011 on non-hepatic applications. Ultraschall Med. 2012;33:33–59. https://doi.org/10.1055/s-0031-1281676.
31. Michels G, Breitkreutz R, Pfister R. Value of lung ultrasound in emergency and intensive care medicine. Dtsch Med Wochenschr. 2014;139(45):2301–7. https://doi.org/10.1055/s-0034-1387309.
32. Gardelli G, Feletti F, Nanni A, et al. Chest ultrasonography in the ICU. Respir Care. 2012;57:773–81. https://doi.org/10.4187/respcare.01743.
33. Lichtenstein DA. Lung ultrasound in the critically ill. Ann Intensive Care. 2014;4:1. https://doi.org/10.1186/2110-5820-4-1.
34. Lichtenstein DA. Lung ultrasound (in the critically ill) superior to CT: the example of lung sliding. Korean J Crit Care Med. 2017;32(1):1–8. https://doi.org/10.4266/kjccm.2016.00955.
35. Armbruster W, Eichholz R, Notheisen T. Lung ultrasound for anesthesia, intensive care and emergency medicine. Anasthesiol Intensivmed Notfallmed Schmerzther. 2019;54(2):108–27. https://doi.org/10.1055/a-0664-5700.
36. Efremov SM, Kuzkov VV, Fot EV, Kirov MY, Ponomarev DN, Lakhin RE, Kokarev EA. Lung ultrasonography and cardiac surgery: a narrative review. Cardiothorac Vasc Anesth. 2020; https://doi.org/10.1053/j.jvca.2020.01.032.
37. Ziskin MC, et al. The comet tail artifact. J Ultrasound Med. 1982;1:1–7. https://doi.org/10.7863/jum.1982.1.1.1.
38. Dietrich CF, Mathis G, Blaivas M, Volpicelli G, Seibel A, Wastl D, Atkinson NS, Cui XW, Fan M, Yi D. Lung B-line artefacts and their use. J Thorac Dis. 8:1356–65. https://doi.org/10.21037/jtd.2016.04.55.
39. Lesser TG. Significance of thoracic and lung ultrasound in thoracic surgery. Ultraschall Med. 2017;38(6):592–610. https://doi.org/10.1055/s-0043-119873.
40. Goffi A, Kruisselbrink R, Volpicelli G. The sound of air: point-of care lung ultrasound in perioperative medicine. Can J Anesth. 2018;65:399–416. https://doi.org/10.1007/s12630-018-1062-x.

41. https://www.degum.de/fileadmin/dokumente/service/Downloads/Poster_A4-Lungenultraschall-protokoll_DEGUM_SGUM_OEGM_V3_06042020_Print_digital_NEU. pdf. Accessed 4 Jan 2020.

42. Lu W, Zhang S, Chen B, Chen J, Xian J, Lin Y, Shan H, Su ZZ. A clinical study of noninvasive assessment of lung lesions in patients with coronavirus disease-19 (COVID-19) by bedside ultrasound. Ultraschall Med. 2020;41(3):300–7. https://doi.org/10.1055/a-1154-8795.

43. Soummer A, Perbet S, Brisson H, Arbelot C, Constantin JM, Lu Q, Rouby JJ, Lung Ultrasound Study Group. Ultrasound assessment of lung aeration loss during a successful weaning trial predicts postextubation distress. Crit Care Med. 2012;40(7):2064–72. https://doi.org/10.1097/CCM.0b013e31824e68ae.

44. Clevert DA, D'Anastasi M, Jung EM. Contrast-enhanced ultrasound and microcirculation: efficiency through dynamics--current developments. Clin Hemorheol Microcirc. 2013;53(1–2):171–86. https://doi.org/10.3233/CH-2012-1584.

45. Clevert DA, Jung EM. Interventional sonography of the liver and kidneys. Radiologe. 2013;53(11):962–73. https://doi.org/10.1007/s00117-012-2459-0.

46. Rübenthaler J, Paprottka KJ, Marcon J, Reiser M, Clevert DA. MRI and contrast enhanced ultrasound (CEUS) image fusion of renal lesions. Clin Hemorheol Microcirc. 2016;64(3):457–66. https://doi.org/10.3233/CH-168116.

47. Zimmermann H, Rübenthaler J, Paprottka P, Paprottka KJ, Reiser M, Clevert DA. Feasability of contrast-enhanced ultrasound with image fusion of CEUS and MS-CT for endovascular grafting in infrarenal abdominal aortic aneurysm in a single patient. Clin Hemorheol Microcirc. 2016;64(4):711–9. https://doi.org/10.3233/CH-168045.

48. Paprottka PM, Zengel P, Cyran CC, Paprottka KJ, Ingrisch M, Nikolaou K, Reiser MF, Clevert DA. Evaluation of multimodality imaging using image fusion with MRI and CEUS in an experimental animal model. Clin Hemorheol Microcirc. 2015;61(2):143–50. https://doi.org/10.3233/CH-151986.

49. Jung EM, Clevert DA. Possibilities of sonographic image fusion: current developments. Radiologe. 2015;55(11):937–48. https://doi.org/10.1007/s00117-015-0025-2.

50. Paprottka PM, Zengel P, Cyran CC, Ingrisch M, Nikolaou K, Reiser MF, Clevert DA. Evaluation of multimodality imaging using image fusion with ultrasound tissue elasticity imaging in an experimental animal model. Clin Hemorheol Microcirc. 2014;57(2):101–10. https://doi.org/10.3233/CH-141821.

51. Clevert DA, Paprottka PM, Helck A, Reiser M, Trumm CG. Image fusion in the management of thermal tumor ablation of the liver. Clin Hemorheol Microcirc. 2012;52(2–4):205–16. https://doi.org/10.3233/CH-2012-1598.

52. Helck A, Notohamiprodjo M, Danastasi M, Meinel F, Reiser M, Clevert DA. Ultrasound image fusion - clinical implementation and potential benefits for monitoring of renal transplants. Clin Hemorheol Microcirc. 2012;52(2–4):179–86. https://doi.org/10.3233/CH-2012-1595.

53. Clevert DA, Helck A, Paprottka PM, Zengel P, Trumm C, Reiser MF. Ultrasound-guided image fusion with computed tomography and magnetic resonance imaging. Clinical utility for imaging and interventional diagnostics of hepatic lesions. Radiologe. 2012;52(1):63–9. https://doi.org/10.1007/s00117-011-2252-5.

54. Clevert DA, Helck A, D'Anastasi M, Gürtler V, Sommer WH, Meimarakis G, Weidenhagen R, Reiser M. Improving the follow up after EVAR by using ultrasound image fusion of CEUS and MS-CT. Clin Hemorheol Microcirc. 2011;49(1–4):91–104. https://doi.org/10.3233/CH-2011-1460.

55. Rennert J, Georgieva M, Schreyer AG, Jung W, Ross C, Stroszczynski C, et al. Image fusion of contrast enhanced ultrasound (CEUS) with computed tomography (CT) or magnetic resonance imaging (MRI) using volume navigation for detection, characterization and planning of therapeutic interventions of liver tumors. Clin Hemorheol Microcirc. 2011;49(1–4):67–81. https://doi.org/10.3233/CH-2011-1458.

56. Bai HX, Hsieh B, Xiong Z, Halsey K, Choi JW, Tran TML, Pan I, Shi LB, Wang DC, Mei J, Jiang XL, Zeng QH, Egglin TK, Hu PF, Agarwal S, Xie F, Li S, Healey T, Atalay MK, Liao

WH. Performance of radiologists in differentiating COVID-19 from viral pneumonia on chest CT. Radiology. 2020;296(2):46–54. https://doi.org/10.1148/radiol.2020200823.

57. Liu J, Feng X, et al. New guidelines for ultrasonic diagnosis of neonatal lung diseases. Chin J Contemp Pediatr. 2019;21(02):105–13.

58. Leech M, Bissett B, Kot M, et al. Lung ultrasound for critical care physiotherapists: a narrative review. Physiother Res Int. 2015;20(2):69–76. https://doi.org/10.1002/pri.1607.

59. Huang Y, Wang S, Liu Y, Zhang Y, Zheng C, Zheng Y, Zhang C, Min W, Zhou H, Yu M, Hu M. A preliminary study on the ultrasonic manifestations of peripulmonary lesions of non-critical novel coronavirus pneumonia (COVID-19). https://ssrn.com/. Accessed 7 May 2021.

60. Blaivas M, DeBehnke D, Phelan MB. Potential errors in the diagnosis of pericardial effusion on trauma ultrasound for penetrating injuries. Acad Emerg Med. 2000;7(11):1261–6. https://doi.org/10.1111/j.1553-2712.2000.tb00472.x.

61. Clevert, Schröder, Sabel, Atemnot und Ultraschall, Bayerisches Ärzteblatt. 2020;204. https://www.bayerisches-aerzteblatt.de/fileadmin/aerzteblatt/ausgaben/2020/05/einzelpdf/BAB_5_2020_204_206.pdf. Accessed 3 May 2020.

62. White paper: lung ultrasound in patients with coronavirus COVID-19 disease. 2020. https://www.siemens-healthineers.com/de/ultrasound/lung-ultrasound-covid-19. Accessed 7 May 2020.

Clinical Covid-19 Lung Imaging

4

Rachel B. Liu and Daniel Vryhof

4.1 Introduction

Lung ultrasound has emerged as an initial imaging modality of choice for diagnosing suspected SARS-CoV-2. Given inconsistencies with swab testing availability, turnaround time delays for results and test variabilities, clinicians have turned to imaging and other laboratory parameters to assist diagnosis. Computed tomography (CT) is the most sensitive modality for diagnosing COVID-19 pneumonia, as high as 97% when compared to reverse-transcription polymerase-chain reaction (RT-PCR) nasal swab tests [1]. However, concerns regarding resource utilization, contamination of fixed suites, infection control requirements and transmission exposure to transport personnel have prevented it from becoming a ubiquitous standard in evaluation of COVID-19 infected patients. The American College of Radiology (ACR) recommended against its use as a first-line diagnostic test [2].

Historically, lung ultrasound has proven useful for pulmonary evaluations during prior global crises such as the 2009 H1N1 influenza pandemic and the 2013 H7N9 avian influenza A epidemic. It has shown large promise in COVID-19 as well, with radiologic severity, progression and resolution of disease on CT mirrored by changes evident using lung ultrasound. Ultrasound may be superior to standard chest

Supplementary Information The online version of this chapter (https://doi.org/10.1007/978-3-030-66614-9_4) contains supplementary material, which is available to authorized users.

R. B. Liu (✉)
Department of Emergency Medicine, Yale School of Medicine, New Haven, CT, USA
e-mail: rachel.liu@yale.edu

D. Vryhof
Department of Emergency Medicine, Columbia University Medical Center, New York Presbyterian Hospital, New York, NY, USA
e-mail: dv2448@cumc.columbia.edu

radiographs particularly early in infection processes [3–5]. Additionally, lung ultrasound is easily repeatable while other imaging modalities are not, and can be deployed at bedside for evaluation of unstable patients.

During the COVID-19 global outbreak, physicians and other health professionals are taking advantage of newer, inexpensive handheld tablet ultrasound devices in an attempt to prevent fomite transmission from larger machines, as these less complex devices are easier to clean. Remote or at-home monitoring has been described, with infected healthcare professionals performing self-assessments of their own or colleagues' lung ultrasounds during quarantine periods. Teleguidance has become more feasible to implement, enhancing remote review capabilities [5–7].

4.2 Findings

Descriptions of COVID-19 lung ultrasound findings include:

- Multifocal, patchy B lines (also referred to as alveolar interstitial edema)
- Thickening of the pleural line or an irregularly appearing pleural line
- Peripheral and bilaterally diffuse but asymmetric locations
- Subpleural consolidations
- Larger lobar consolidations with air bronchograms
- Rarely, pleural effusion

Nomenclature with lung ultrasound may be confusing, with multiple terms used to describe variations in similar concepts. Lung ultrasound artifacts were discovered and initially coined by Lichtenstein in his BLUE protocol [8], and have been further clarified since due to heterogeneity in appearance [9]. B lines refer to vertical, "laser-like" hyperechoic lines which begin at the pleural line and extend along the full field of view, moving with pleural movement (Fig. 4.1). Lung fields are considered positive for interstitial fluid if more than three B lines are present, and more severe disease is indicated by coalescing of multiple individual B lines into cohesive formations. Subclassifications of these B line appearances in COVID-19 have been described as "waterfall" or "white lung" signs indicating diffuse B lines which are fused and potentially more fixed than in other disease processes (Figs. 4.2 and 4.3) [4, 10]. Recently, Volpicelli and Gargani identified a B line appearance which could indicate the early development of COVID-19 ground glass opacities as "light beams." These are described as "shining band-form" artifacts that arise from large areas of normal-appearing pleural lines that disappear and reappear with respiration, through which A lines (normal) can be visualized. The authors suggest that presence of this appearance correlates with a high probability of COVID-19 diagnosis [11].

Others describe a thickened pleural line with a rough or irregular, interrupted appearance (Fig. 4.4) [6, 10–12]. This is due to thickening and edema of affected interstitial tissues and pleura, with occasional localized pleural effusions adjacent to the lesions. A noncontiguous appearance of the pleural line may also be due to small subpleural consolidations, which have varied shapes and sizes. Subpleural

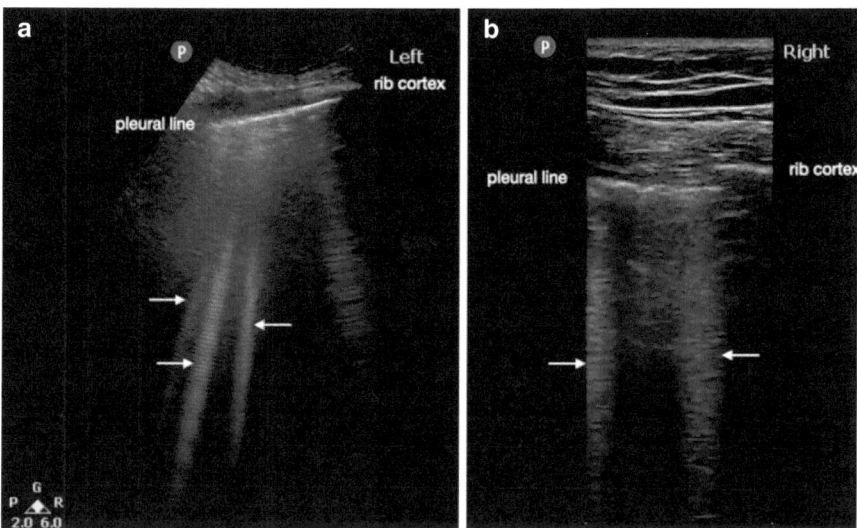

Fig. 4.1 Examples of B lines. (**a**) Scan performed with a curvilinear transducer (**b**) Scan performed with a linear transducer. B lines are indicated by arrows. B lines arise from the pleural line and extend through the full field of view, erasing normally existing horizontal A lines. B lines move with pleural line movement, as seen in the Extra Supplementary Materials (B lines video)

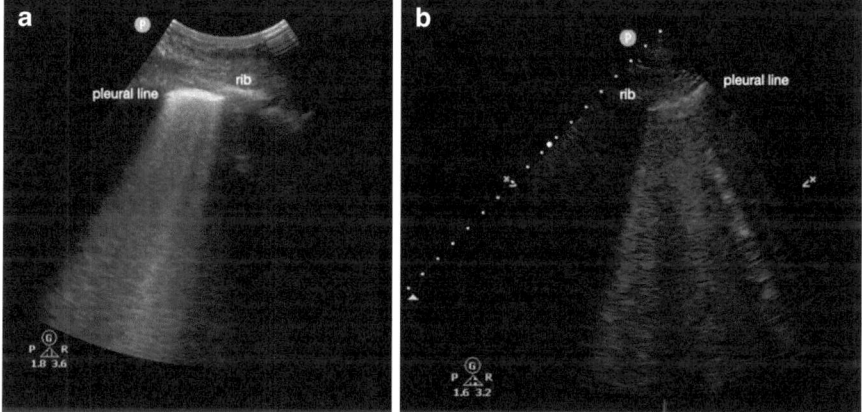

Fig. 4.2 Diffuse, more coalescent B lines. (**a**) Scan performed with a curvilinear transducer, with thickening of the pleural line and a diffuse pattern of B lines, which some refer to as a waterfall appearance. (**b**) Scan performed with a phased array transducer, showing multiple B lines which are starting to fuse. Dynamic images are demonstrated in the Extra Supplementary Materials (Coalescent B lines Video)

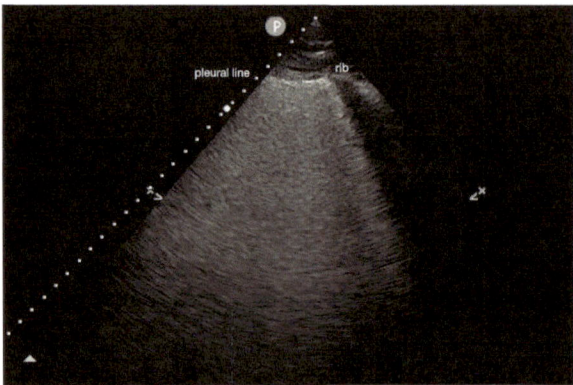

Fig. 4.3 Saturation of B lines, "white lung" appearance. Image obtained using a phased array transducer. Notice how the full field is covered with a large, wide pattern of coalescent B lines which cannot be visually separated. This indicates interstitial saturation and would cause severe shortness of breath. Corresponds to Extra Supplementary Materials

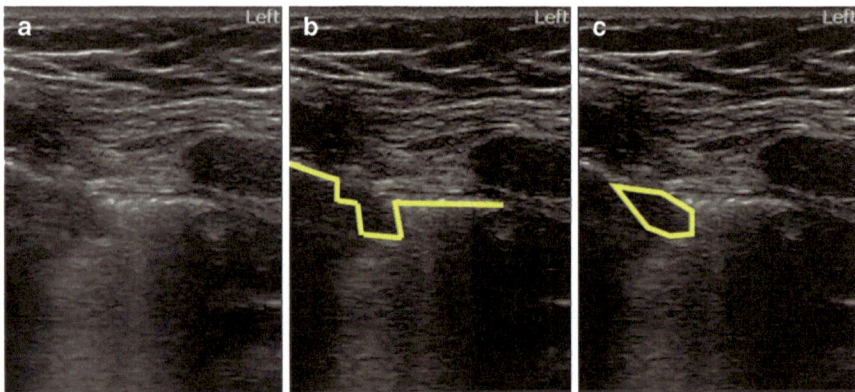

Fig. 4.4 Irregular Pleural Line caused by a subpleural consolidation. (**a**) B-mode view of a non-contiguous, irregular, nonlinear pleural line caused by a subpleural consolidation (the hypoechoic circular structure underneath the pleural line. (**b**) Illustration of the pleural irregularity. (**c**) Illustration of the subpleural consolidation. Corresponds to Extra Supplementary Materials (Subpleural Consolidation Video)

consolidations may demonstrate air bronchograms within them, and color flow Doppler may show poor flow to these regions. This may be important, as consolidations caused by inflammation typically show good blood flow, indicating reassuring prognoses. However, poor flow may indicate an inability to develop microvessel exchange due to the rapid progression of disease in COVID-19 [10], or presence of peripheral microangiopathic lung infarction [13].

These findings are not specific to COVID-19 and are similar to other viral infections or lung conditions. Specificity for COVID-19 is increased with a noncontiguous multifocal pattern of B lines, present in some areas while spared in others, leading to "patchwork" clusters of disease. A more uniform appearance may suggest other pathologies [4, 5, 11]. Numerous studies demonstrate that in COVID-19, findings are initially most prominent in the posterior and inferior lung fields [3–5, 10].

4.3 Approaches

For general lung ultrasound, the BLUE protocol identified 3 areas for scanning a hemithorax (anterior, lateral and posterolateral), with each area further subdivided into upper and lower halves. This produces 6 zones per chest wall side, for a total of 12 zones when imaging the whole thorax. This method has been used in some scoring methods which compare lung ultrasound to CT correlation [4]. Soldati et al. used a 14 zone approach performed in sitting patients to establish a lung ultrasound scoring system specific to COVID-19 patients. This includes 7 zones per hemithorax. These were defined as 3 posterior views along the paravertebral line, 2 lateral views along the midaxillary line, and 2 anterior views along the midclavicular line. Obtaining posterior views may be difficult in recumbent patients (e.g., intubated patients), and they identified the lower posterolateral point as a high-yield area for evaluation [6]. In a letter, the same authors advocated for a 16 zone approach as ideal. Others are in favor of a simpler 4–6 zone approach [3, 13]. Due to prominence of findings in the postero-inferior lung fields, these zones may be of primary focus early in the infection before diffuse progression.

Convex array and linear transducers are primarily used to evaluate lung spaces and pleura. Either may be used with COVID-19 patients, but curvilinear transducers are generally favored as they can evaluate both pleural and parenchymal areas with a larger surface area, allowing quick evaluation of the whole chest wall [11, 15]. Linear transducers may be used for heightened definition of the pleural line and delineation of subpleural consolidations [14], particularly in the lung periphery. Low frequency microconvex and phased array transducers have been used as well.

Traditionally, the probe is placed perpendicular (longitudinally) to each rib and intercostal space surface, visualizing rib shadows at the cephalad and caudal fields of view. This covers maximal surface area within a single scan as multiple intercostal spaces can be imaged simultaneously [15]. However, some advocate for the probe to be oriented transversely or obliquely (in parallel with rib direction) to interrogate a wider surface of lung pleura or parenchyma [4, 14]. Using a combination of these orientations with continuous multidirectional sliding, sweeping and rotating of the transducer in a "lawnmower" technique will allow thorough lung evaluation. A full lung ultrasound assessment takes 5 to 8 min for completion by an experienced sonologist [4].

Table 4.1 Examples of scoring systems

Authors	Probe type	Zones	Scoring
Tan G, et al. (*ICU physicians*)	Convex array	10 zones, 5 per side • Anterior upper • Anterior lower • Phrenic point • Posterolateral alveolar (PLAPS) • Posterior Based on BLUE protocol	0—normal pleura 1—thickened or irregular pleura (>0.5 mm) 2—blurred pleural line 3—discontinuous line 0—no B line 1—B lines <3 2—B lines <4 3—fused B lines 4—consolidation 0—no complications 4—am line 4—pneumothorax or empyema 4—pleural effusion
Lu W, et al. (*1 ultrasound physician*)	Convex array then linear transducer	12 zones, 6 per side • Anterior upper • Anterior lower • Lateral upper • Lateral lower • Posterior upper • Posterior lower Based on BLUE protocol	0—normal pleura 1—B lines >3 2—coalesced B lines 3—consolidation Severity: 0, none 1–7, mild 8–18, moderate >19, severe
Soldati G, et al. (*multiple specialties*)	Convex Array	14 zones, 7 per side • Basal, paravertebral • Middle, paravertebral • Upper, paravertebral • Basal, midaxillary • Upper, midaxillary • Basal, midclavicular • Upper, midclavicular	0—normal pleura 1—pleural line indented 2—pleural line broken (small consolidations) 3—white lung with or without larger consolidation Severity thresholds not described
Volpicelli G, et al. (*Emergency and ICU setting*)	Convex array	10 zones • Anterior chest • Lateral chest • Lateral chest, inferior in oblique view • Posterior chest between the scapula and spine • Posterior chest below the scapula	0—normal pleura 1—multiple separated B lines 2—coalescent B lines or light beam 3—consolidation Percentage of pathologic presence assigned and averaged Used to quantify an aeration score, and then assess dynamic changes in aeration by reassigning new scores to re-aerated areas

4.4 Clinical Integration

Prior scoring systems have shown value for acute respiratory distress syndrome in the intensive care unit (ICU). A few specific scoring systems have been proposed to aid determination of COVID-19 disease severity, in conjunction with clinical parameters (Table 4.1). They possess similar elements, but the clinical value of these scoring systems and their influence in determining patient dispositions, treatments or admission levels of care has yet to be elucidated. Similarly, their roles in predicting patient deterioration or readiness for de-escalation require further research. However, a patient's severity of disease may be proportional to the amount of lung parenchyma that exhibit ground glass changes, and early quantification of lung involvement may be beneficial. Volpicelli reports that using lung ultrasound findings in dorsal areas prompts decisions to prone patients who are receiving higher forms of ventilation, and the scoring system the authors developed may be used to monitor dynamic changes in aeration that could aid recruitment and ventilation strategies. Tan et al. developed a scoring system which helped differentiate between COVID-19 pneumonia and community acquired pneumonia, which showed larger and more circumscribed consolidations with associated pleural effusions in the latter illness [16].

Others have proposed algorithms that use lung ultrasound for triage, cohorting, and admission criteria [11, 17]. While a discharge and follow up plan for patients with both mild symptoms and mild findings on lung ultrasound, or an admission plan for severe disease with significant lung ultrasound findings is self-explanatory, the impact of lung ultrasound for moderate COVID-19 disease needs to be explored. For example, even if a patient demonstrates significant lung ultrasound findings, it would still be reasonable for a clinically well appearing person to be discharged with a close follow-up plan. Those with more worrisome clinical signs (significant hypoxia or tachypnea) may warrant admission, even if their initial lung ultrasound findings appear mild. Completely negative lung ultrasound findings in COVID-19 suspected patients prompts exploration for other extrapulmonary diagnoses (such as cardiac manifestations), and this is a key usage. As CT findings map disease progression and chronology, lung ultrasound findings can similarly be used to match a patient's disease timeline.

Mongodi et al. compared imaging resource utilization during COVID-19 with a historical time period, and found that implementing an ultrasound-based approach to imaging decreased the number of chest radiographs and CTs used for acute respiratory failure patients during the height of the pandemic [18]. A study using an emergency room patient cohort found that anterior upper and lower B lines were independently associated with development of acute respiratory distress syndrome (ARDS) in COVID-19 patients, as well as with ICU admission [3]. Given that dorsal changes may appear earlier, progression of B lines to become evident in anterior zones (anatomically higher positions) even without evaluation of posterior areas could indicate severe disease. Additionally, lung ultrasound findings may predict which phenotype of COVID-19 a patient has, although the impact of this to clinical care is unknown [13]. It may be possible to differentiate B lines caused by COVID-19 from B lines caused by fluid overload or cardiogenic pulmonary edema. As such, specialist services have applied lung and cardiac ultrasound to treatment algorithms for their patients, such as determining safety for dialysis treatment [15].

Overall, more large-scale research is needed to assess the performance of lung ultrasound algorithms or scoring systems in predicting patient course, ventilation strategies, effectiveness of maneuvers like prone positioning, and applicability to the different phenotypes of COVID-19 [13]. These purposes advocate for patient monitoring via serial lung ultrasound performance, which may suggest patient deterioration or treatment non-response via development of superimposed bacterial pneumonia or increasing B lines. These could trigger titration of positive end-expiratory pressure and addition of other recruitment aides. Likewise, resolution of B lines indicates patient improvement, and may suggest that attempts to wean respiratory supports would be successful [5, 11].

4.5 Test Characteristics

While no author recommends that ultrasound can be used as a CT replacement, bedside lung ultrasound has shown moderate agreement with CT findings in both European and Chinese patient studies. Nouvenne et al. found a significant positive correlation of lung ultrasound with CT findings on Spearman correlation ($r = 0.65$, $p < 0.001$) and a negative correlation with oxygen saturation ($r = -0.66$, $p < 0.001$) upon hospital admission of COVID-19 patients [19]. Lu et al. showed similar, with moderate Kappa agreement between lung ultrasound and CT findings of 30 COVID-19 patients ($k = 0.529$, $p < 0.05$) [4]. This suggests that lung ultrasound may be a reliable first-line imaging study, comparable to CT. As with all ultrasound, it is an operator dependent modality and areas of disease may be missed if not scanned adequately.

Bar et al. found lung ultrasound odds ratios that were independently associated with COVID-19 ARDS development and ICU admission (anterior upper zone B lines >3 = 1.52 OR, inferior thickened pleura = 1.73 OR, lower zone consolidation = 2.39 OR, posterolateral thickened pleura = 1.97 OR). Mortality was not associated with these variables [3].

The sensitivity for lung ultrasound in categories of no disease, mild, moderate and severe COVID-19 disease increases with severity (33.3%, 68.8, 77.8%, and 100% respectively). Specificity for these same categories is high (100%, 85.7%, 76.2%, and 92.9% respectively). Positive predictive values range from 50–100%, with lower values associated with more severe disease. Negative predictive values range from 70.6–100%, with highest values for the no disease or severe disease categories. Diagnostic accuracy ranges from 76.7–93.3%, again with highest values seen for the no disease or severe disease categories [4]. Lung ultrasound shows higher sensitivity for lesions near the pleura (peripheral), and may underestimate consolidations located away from the pleura. Comparatively in H1N1 disease, lung ultrasound demonstrated a 94% sensitivity, 89% specificity, 86% positive predictive value, and a 96% negative predictive value that outperformed chest radiographs [5].

These parameters of lung ultrasound in COVID-19 appear similar and suggest that it can be used for risk stratification of suspected patients.

4.6 Summary

Lung ultrasound has repeatedly shown effectiveness in the diagnosis and monitoring of viral pneumonias in pandemic or epidemic situations. The usefulness of bedside ultrasound has been firmly established with the COVID-19 pandemic, particularly in reducing workforce exposure in such a virulent disease. Although further research with large populations are needed to solidify the role of lung ultrasound in clinical management of patients and its influence on patient outcomes, the benefits in respiratory monitoring, guiding treatment decisions, and predicting escalations or de-escalations of care have been well described. It is incorporated into multiorgan point-of-care ultrasound to simultaneously examine both pulmonary and extrapulmonary etiologies of COVID-19 symptoms. Its test characteristics appear reasonable for continued use by trained, experienced personnel. These descriptions will serve as a basis for future COVID-19 care, as further waves are anticipated. The insertion of lung ultrasound in triage algorithms serves as a template for future respiratory pandemics.

References

1. Ai T, Yang Z, Hou H, Zhan C, Chen C, Lv W, et al. Correlation of chest CT and RT-PCR testing in coronavirus disease 2019 (COVID-19) in China: a report of 1014 cases. Radiology. 2020:2006–42.
2. American College of Radiology (ACR): ACR Recommendations for the use of Chest Radiography and Computed Tomography (CT) for Suspected COVID-19 Infection. 2020. https://www.acr.org/Advocacy-and-Economics/ACR-Position-Statements/Recommendations-for-Chest-Radiography-and-CT-for-Suspected-COVID19-Infection. Accessed 6 June 2020.
3. Bar S, Lecourtois A, Diouf M, Goldberg E, Bourbon C, Arnaud E, et al. The association of lung ultrasound images with COVID-19 infection in an emergency room cohort. Anaesthesia. 2020;75(12):1620–5.
4. Lu W, Zhang S, Chen B, Chen J, Xian J, Lin Y, et al. A clinical study of noninvasive assessment of lung lesions in patients with coronavirus disease (COVID-19) by bedside ultrasound. Ultraschall Med. 2020;41(3):300–7.
5. Convissar D, Gibson LE, Berra L, Bittner EA, Change MG. Application of lung ultrasound during the COVID-19 pandemic: a narrative review. Anesth Analg. 2020;131(2):345–50.
6. Soldati G, Smargiassi A, Inchingolo R, Buonsenso D, Perrone T, Briganti DF, et al. Proposal for international standardization of the use of lung ultrasound for patients with COVID-19. J Ultrasound Med. 2020;39(7):1413–9.
7. Liu RB, Tayal VS, Panebianco NL, Tung-Chen Y, Nagdev A, Shah S, et al. Ultrasound on the frontlines of COVID-19: a report from an international webinar. Acad Emerg Med. 2020;27(6):523–6.
8. Lichtenstein DA, Meziere GA. Relevance of lung ultrasound in the diagnosis of acute respiratory failure: the BLUE protocol. Chest. 2008;134:117–25.
9. Lichtenstein DA. Lung ultrasound in the critically ill. Ann Intensive Care. 2014;4(1):1.

10. Huang Y, Wang S, Liu Y. A preliminary study on the ultrasonic manifestations of peripulmonary lesions of non-critical novel coronavirus pneumonia (COVID-19). Soc Sci Res Netw. 2020. https://papers.ssrn.com/sol3/papers.cfm?abstract_id=3544750. Accessed 6 June 2020.
11. Volpicelli G, Lamorte A, Villen T. What's new in lung ultrasound during the COVID-19 pandemic. Intensive Care Med. 2020;46(7):1445–8.
12. Peng QY, Wang XT, Zhang LN. Findings of lung ultrasonography of novel coronavirus pneumonia during the 2019 – 2020 epidemic. Intensive Care Med. 2020;46(5):849–50.
13. Denault AY, Delisle S, Canty D, Royse A, Royse C, Cid Serra X, et al. A proposed lung ultrasound and phenotypic algorithm for the care of COVID-19 patients with acute respiratory failure. Can J Anesth. 2020;21:1–12.
14. Soldati G, Smargiassi A, Inchingolo R, Buonsenso D, Perrone T, Briganti DF, et al. Is there a role for lung ultrasound during the COVID-19 pandemic? J Ultrasound Med. 2020;39(7):1459–62.
15. Viera ALS, Junior JM, Bastos MG. Role of point of care ultrasound during the COVID-19 pandemic: our recommendations in the management of dialytic patients. Ultrasound J. 2020;12:30.
16. Tan G, Lian X, Zhu Z, Wang Z, Huang F, Zhang Y, et al. Use of lung ultrasound to differentiate coronavirus disease 2019 (COVID-19) pneumonia from community-acquired pneumonia. Ultrasound Med Biol. 2020;46(10):2651–8.
17. Guarracino F, Vetrugno L, Forfori F, Corradi F, Orso D, Bertini P, et al. Lung, heart, vascular, and diaphragm ultrasound examination of COVID-19 patients: a comprehensive approach. J Cardiothorac Vasc Anesth. 2021;35(6):1866–74.
18. Mongodi S, Orlando A, Arisi E, Tavazzi G, Santangelo E, Canva L, et al. Lung ultrasound in patients with acute respiratory failure reduces conventional imaging and health care provider exposure to COVID-19. Ultrasound Med Biol. 2020;46(8):2090–3.
19. Nouvenne A, Zani MD, Milanese G, Parise A, Baciarello M, Bignami EG, et al. Lung ultrasound in COVID-19 pneumonia: correlations with chest CT on hospital admission. Respiration. 2020;99(7):617–24.

Pediatric Covid-19 Lung Ultrasound

5

Danilo Buonsenso and Cristina De Rose

5.1   Introduction

Initially described in China in December 2019, severe acute respiratory syndrome coronavirus 2 (SARS-CoV-2) has spread all over the world, infecting more than one million people and causing thousands of deaths [1]. Humans of all age groups are susceptible, including the youngest. Although currently pediatric coronavirus disease 19 (COVID-19) appears to be less severe compared with the adult form, children are by no means spared. Several case series [2–5] have documented that COVID-19 can affect children of all ages, from newborns to adolescents [6].

Disease severity can be classified, adapting a previous published classification[2], based on predefined criteria (Table 5.1) [7].

COVID-19 pneumonia has also been described in asymptomatic or pauci-symptomatic children [2–4]. However, in rare cases, children can be severely affected, and clinical manifestations may differ from adults. In April of 2020, reports emerged from the United Kingdom of a presentation in children similar to incomplete Kawasaki disease (KD) or toxic shock syndrome [8, 9]. Since then, there have been increasing reports of similarly affected children in other parts of the world [10–16].

The syndrome has been termed multisystem inflammatory syndrome in children (MIS-C; also referred to as pediatric multisystem inflammatory syndrome [PMIS], pediatric inflammatory multisystem syndrome temporally associated with SARS-CoV-2 [PIMS-TS], pediatric hyperinflammatory syndrome, or pediatric hyperinflammatory shock).

D. Buonsenso (✉) · C. De Rose
Department of Woman and Child Health and Public Health, Fondazione Policlinico Universitario A. Gemelli IRCCS, Università Cattolica del Sacro Cuore, Rome, Italy
e-mail: danilo.buonsenso@policlinicogemelli.it

Table 5.1 Disease severity [2, 7]

Asymptomatic: All the following must be present
1. No signs or symptoms
2. AND negative chest X-ray
3. AND absence of criteria for other cases
Mild: Any of the following (AND absence of criteria for more severe cases)
1. Symptoms of upper respiratory tract infection
2. AND absence of pneumonia at chest X-ray
Moderate: All the following (AND absence of criteria for more severe cases)
1. Cough AND (sick appearing OR pneumonia at chest X-ray)
Severe: Any of the following (AND absence of criteria as for critical case)
2. Oxygen saturation <92%
3. OR difficult breathing or other signs of severe respiratory distress (apnea, gasping, head nodding)
4. OR need for any respiratory support
Critical: Any of the following
1. Patient in ICU
2. OR intubated
3. OR multiorgan failure
4. OR shock, encephalopathy, myocardial injury or heart failure, coagulation dysfunction, acute kidney injury

Adapted from Dong et al. [2]

While the incidence of MIS-C is unknown, it appears to be a rare complication of COVID-19 in children.

Many children with MIS-C meet criteria for complete or incomplete Kawasaki disease (KD) (Table 5.2) [8, 10, 11, 14, 17–19]. However, the epidemiology differs from that of classic KD. Most MIS-C cases have occurred in older children and adolescents who were previously healthy. Black and Hispanic children may be disproportionally affected. By contrast, classic KD typically affects infants and young children and has a higher incidence in East Asia and in children of Asian descent. The epidemiology of MIS-C also differs from that of acute COVID-19 illness in children, which tends to be most severe in infants <1 year of age and in children with underlying health problems [10–12, 17–19].

5.2 Role of Imaging in Pediatrics

Although a nasopharyngeal swab is required for a definitive etiologic diagnosis of 2019 novel coronavirus disease, this test has limitations, particularly because of its low sensitivity [20]. For this reason, several authors have suggested the use of chest computed tomography (CT) not only for diagnosis of COVID-19 pneumonia, but also as a screening tool for the diagnosis of COVID-19 infection in epidemic settings, as CT has been reported to have better diagnostic sensitivity than nasopharyngeal swab [21]. Conversely, Rubin et al. [22] suggested an appropriate use of imaging, selecting those patients that might benefit from the adjunctive information contained in images. However, CT scan should not be routinely used in specific age

Table 5.2 Clinical manifestations of COVID-19-associated multisystem inflammatory syndrome in children and adolescents [8, 10, 11, 14, 17–19]

Presenting symptoms	Frequency (%)
Persistent fevers (median duration 4 days)	100
Gastrointestinal symptoms (abdominal pain, vomiting, diarrhea)	60–100
Rash	52–76
Conjunctivitis	45–81
Mucous membrane involvement	29–76
Neurocognitive symptoms (headache, lethargy, confusion)	29–58
Respiratory symptoms (tachypnea, labored breathing)	21–65
Swollen hands/feet	16
Sore throat	10
Clinical findings	
Shock	50–80
Criteria for complete Kawasaki disease met	21–64
Myocardial dysfunction (by echocardiogram or elevated troponin/BNP)	51–100
Acute respiratory failure requiring noninvasive or invasive ventilation	43–52
Acute kidney injury	21–70
Serositis (small pleural, pericardial, and ascitic effusions)	22–57
Acute hepatic failure	21
Laboratory findings	
Abnormal blood cell counts	
Lymphocytopenia	80–95
Neutrophilia	80–90
Mild anemia	70
Thrombocytopenia	31–80
Elevated inflammatory markers	
C-reactive protein	90–100
Erythrocyte sedimentation rate	80
D-dimer	80–100
Fibrinogen	90–100
Ferritin	55–76
Procalcitonin	80–95
Interleukin-6	80–100
Elevated cardiac markers	
Troponin	68–95
BNP or NT-pro-BNP	78–100
Hypoalbuminemia	73–95
Mildly elevated liver enzymes	60–70
Elevated lactate dehydrogenase	56–60
Hypertriglyceridemia	70
Imaging findings	
Echocardiogram	
Depressed LV function	29–58
Coronary artery dilation/aneurysm	14–48
Other findings can include mitral regurgitation and pericardial effusion	–

(continued)

Table 5.2 (continued)

Presenting symptoms	Frequency (%)
Chest radiograph	
Normal in many patients	–
Abnormal findings included small pleural effusions, patchy consolidations, focal consolidation, and atelectasis	–
Chest CT and/or lung ultrasound	
Findings generally similar to those on chest radiograph	–
A few patients had nodular ground-glass opacification	–
Abdominal imaging (ultrasound and/or CT)	
Findings are nonspecific, including free fluid, ascites, bowel and mesenteric inflammation, including terminal ileitis, mesenteric adenopathy/adenitis, and pericholecystic edema	–

COVID-19 coronavirus disease 2019, *BNP* brain natriuretic peptide, *LV* left ventricular, *CT* computed tomography

groups, such as pregnant women [23] and children [24]. Moreover, COVID-19 has become a global disease, logistic difficulties or unavailability of CT scan in low and medium resource settings must be considered. On the other hand, chest X-ray does not have sufficient sensitivity and specificity for detecting COVID-19 pneumonia to be considered as an alternative tool to CT scan. In this context, the evidences have indicated the usefulness of lung ultrasound (LUS) in detecting COVID-19 pneumonia [25–27]. In particular, both Chinese [28] and Italian [29, 30] task forces on the use of LUS in COVID-19 have provided the physical bases and LUS patterns in COVID-19 patients, suggesting that LUS can be a useful tool to diagnose and monitor COVID-19 pneumonia.

The finding that LUS is able to detect COVID-19 pneumonia in children has clinical implications [7, 24, 31, 32].

The Chinese Task Force for Paediatric COVID-19 proposed a severity classification, defining children as asymptomatic, mild, moderate, severe or critical cases [2].

In particular, the "moderate" stage is based on clinical criteria (pneumonia with fever and cough, in the absence of signs of hypoxemia) and/or radiologic criteria, as "some cases may have no clinical signs and symptoms, but chest CT shows lung lesions, which are subclinical" [2].

In fact, in all the large series of pediatric COVID-19 described in China [2–4] the authors routinely used CT scan to determine the severity of the disease. This has caused clinicians and researchers from the rest of the world to overuse CT scan in children, even when they are asymptomatic or pauci-symptomatic. However, there is no evidence that diagnosis and treatment decisions based on CT scans improve outcomes in pediatric COVID-19 infection. Moreover, although chest CT scans improve diagnostic accuracy, doing these scans in children comes with disadvantages, such as high costs, the need for sedation, and radiation exposure.

In fact, international guidelines state that history and examination are the main determinants of pneumonia severity and level of care, reserving imaging to compromised children requiring admission on clinical grounds [33]. Importantly, the large number of asymptomatic and mild pediatric cases of COVID-19 described confirms that radiologic imaging should not be routinely used [2–5].

Thanks to the already proven accuracy of LUS in detecting pediatric pneumonia of any ethology [34–38] and to light of the studies performed for which lung CT scan is not routinely indicated in patients with suspected COVID-19 and mild-moderate clinical features unless they are at risk for disease progression [22, 24], point-of-care tools such as LUS have become fundamental in diagnosing and monitoring COVID-19 pneumonia, particularly in children, who usually have milder manifestations of COVID-19. This reduces unnecessary radiation/sedation in children and exposure of health care workers to SARS-CoV-2 at the same time.

5.3 How to Perform Pediatric Lung Ultrasound in the Time of COVID-19

The staff safety in the airway management of patients with 2019 novel coronavirus disease (COVID-19) must be ensured from the patient's first assessment. In fact, maintaining the safety of the doctor, who meets many people during his daily activity, avoids the spread of the disease to other patients and the possible creation of new epidemic outbreaks. On the other hand, all health care workers are asked to minimize the use of personal protective devices to prevent their shortage. Although, the breathing manifestations of COVID-19 cases in children are generally less severe than those of adult patients [2–4, 7], while waiting for the result of the nasal/pharyngeal swab for COVID-19, children with fever and respiratory symptoms do still need to be seen and differential diagnosis with other known viral or bacterial respiratory infections remains pivotal. It can be based on the clinical and laboratory data and LUS findings. In this contest, in fact, the use of tools such as a stethoscope and radiological devices, can cause the contamination of the medical devices and nosocomial spreading of the virus leading al the contagion of healthcare workers (from doctor to nurse to radiology technicians) and already hospitalized patients who have a higher risk of developing severe COVID-19. In this regard, in 2016, Copetti highlighted how lung ultrasound could have several advantages compared with the use of the stethoscope, to the extent that it could be replaced [39]. His famous article entitled "Is lung ultrasound the stethoscope of the new millennium? Definitely yes" was visionary in 2016 and now, in this historical period, very pertinent. The use of ultrasound is essential in the safe management of the COVID-19 out breaks, since it can allow the concomitant execution of clinical examination and lung imaging at the bedside by the same doctor [31, 40].

In the setting of COVID-19, wireless probe and tablets represent the most appropriate ultrasound equipment. These devices can easily be wrapped in single-use plastic covers reducing the risk of contamination and making easy the sterilization procedures [29, 31, 40]. In case of unavailability of these devices, portable machines dedicated to the exclusive use of COVID-19 patients can be used, although maximum care for sterilization is necessary. In these cases, probe and keyboard covers are anyway suggested, and sterilization procedures necessary following last recommendations [41].

Two different ways of performing lung ultrasound for the evaluation of children with suspected COVID-19 have been introduced. The first based on the use of lung ultrasound by one pediatrician and another assistant wearing the standard personal protections as per World Health Organization (WHO) indications [42]. The second method aims to reduce both the number of operators and the use of personal protective devices and it provides that only one pediatrician is in contact with the patient suspected/positive for COVID-19 [31, 40].

The stethoscope is not used because it is more difficult to have specific covers and there is a higher probability to mistakenly touch either the ocular or the oral mucosa with it. Lung auscultation is therefore substituted by lung visualization with the ultrasound.

These approaches have several advantages, since the same evaluating clinician can visit the patient, perform blood tests or insert intravenous lines if required, and obtain lung images with portable devices at the same time, without to move the child from the consultation room to the radiology room.

In this way, guaranteeing both the patients "rights to be evaluated according to the highest standards of care and, at the same time, the healthcare workers" safety is guaranteed and the minimal use of safety devices.

5.3.1   Ultrasonography Procedure 1 [40]

The pediatrician, wearing the standard personal protections as per WHO indications [42], prepare the ultrasound pocket device, which comprises a wireless probe and a tablet. The probe and tablet are placed in two separate single-use plastic covers (Fig. 5.1). No other medical devices are used. When the two operators enter the isolation room, the pediatrician uses the probe and does the lung ultrasound, the assistant holds the tablet and freezes and stores the images, touching neither the patient nor the surrounding materials. After the procedure, in a dedicated area, the operators easily remove the probe and tablet from the covers, simply letting them slip onto clean towels, where the devices are further sterilized.

Fig. 5.1 The ultrasound pocket device: the probe and tablet are placed in two separate single-use plastic covers

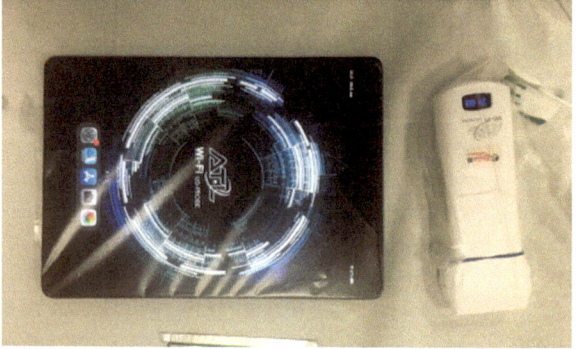

5.3.2 Ultrasonography Procedure 2 [31]

One of the pediatricians prepares the ultrasound pocket device, which comprises a wireless transducer and a tablet. The transducer is placed in single-use plastic covers or a glove sealed with plaster.

Operator 1, wearing the standard personal protections as per World Health Organization indications [42] according to the single situation, enters the isolation room with the wireless transducer and performs the LUS examination. Operator 2 remains outside the room with the tablet communicating with the operator 1 in order to optimize the quality of images. He helps Operator 1 to properly place the probe perpendicularly, obliquely and parallel to the ribs in the anterior, lateral and posterior thorax, so as to perform ultrasound scans in the longitudinal plane and transversal plane. The two operators communicate continuously, giving feedback, on the explored lung fields. Operator 2 is responsible for freezing and storing images/videos (Fig. 5.2). This procedure can reduce the operator dependence of US, since the operators are blinded to each other.

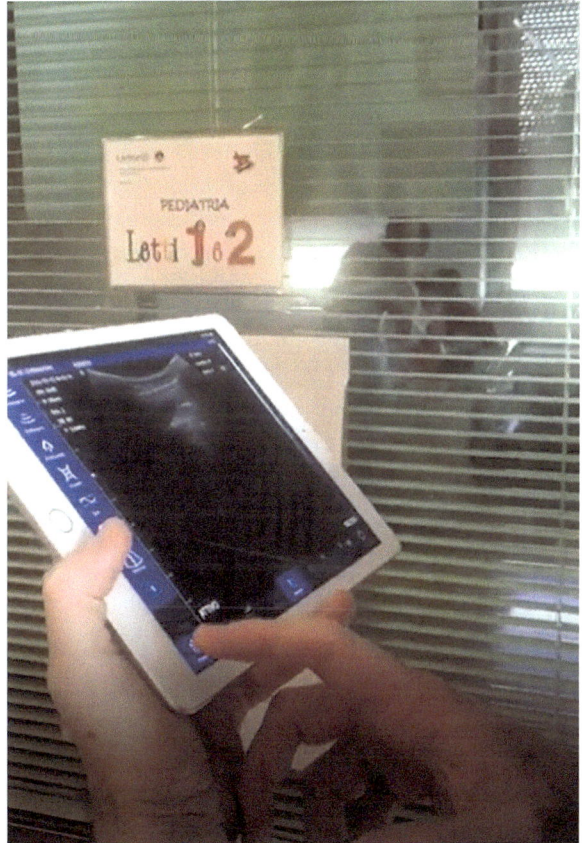

Fig. 5.2 Ultrasonography procedure 2: Operator 2, with the tablet training outsider the room, helps Operator 1 to perform lung ultrasound in order to optimize the quality of images; he is responsible for freezing and storing images/videos. The two operators communicate continuously, giving feedback, on the explored lung fields

At the end of the procedure, only the transducer needs to be sterilized in a dedicated area and put into a new sterile plastic bag.

In both cases, the two operators will follow an agreed, tested, and standardized images acquisition protocol [29].

5.4   Ultrasonography Technique [29]

Fourteen areas (three posterior, two lateral, and two anterior) should be scanned for patient along the lines here indicated. Lung ultrasound should be performed scans in the longitudinal plane and transversal plane. In younger children, uncooperative, scans need to be intercostal as to cover the widest surface possible with one scan.

Examining position can be supine, prone or sitting position to evaluate posterior regions, whichever provides a position of comfort and allows for a complete examination.

Standard sequence of evaluations is proposed using landmarks on chest anatomic lines. Echographic scans can be identified with a progressive numbering starting from right posterior basal regions:

1. Right basal on paravertebral line above the curtain sign
2. Right middle on paravertebral line at the inferior angle of shoulder blade
3. Right upper on paravertebral line at spine of shoulder blade
4. Left basal on paravertebral line above the curtain sign
5. Left middle on paravertebral line at the inferior angle of shoulder blade
6. Left upper on paravertebral line at spine of shoulder blade
7. Right basal on mid-axillary line below the internipple line
8. Right upper on mid-axillary line above the internipple line
9. Left basal on mid-axillary line below the internipple line
10. Left upper on mid-axillary line above the internipple line
11. Right basal on mid-clavicular line below the internipple line
12. Right upper on mid-clavicular line above the internipple line
13. Left basal on mid-clavicular line below the internipple line
14. Left upper on mid-clavicular line above the internipple line

Although mild-moderate cases of COVID-19 pneumonia are much more frequent among the pediatric population, in case of performance of LUS in critical care settings (such as patients on invasive ventilation) and for patients that are not able to maintain sitting position, the posterior areas might be difficult to be evaluated. In these cases, the operator should try to have a partial view of the posterior basal areas, currently considered a "hot-area" for COVID-19, and however, start echographic assessment from landmark number [7].

The appropriate transducers and frequencies vary with the size of the patient. Neonates and small infants are easily examined with high-frequency linear transducers, whereas older children and adolescents require lower-frequency transducers.

5.4.1 Other Specific Indications for the Images Acquisition Protocol

- Use single focal point modality (no multifocusing), setting the focal point on the pleura line. Employing a single focal point, and setting it at the right location, has the benefit to optimize the beam shape for sensing the lung surface. At focus, the beam has the smallest width as is therefore set to best respond to the smallest details.
- Keep the mechanical index (MI) low (start from 0.7 and reduce it further if allowed by the visual findings).
- Avoid as much as possible saturation phenomena, control gain and diminish MI if needed (see example of lung ultrasound images in the figures). Saturation phenomena occurs, e.g., when the signal strength of the echo signals is too high for the receiving electronics to be converted into electrical signals conserving a linear relation with the pressure amplitude. This has the effect of distorting the signals, and produces images where the dynamics of the actual signal is lost. The visual appearance of this phenomenon is the presence of areas which are completely white. In this case, it is therefore not possible to appreciate local variations in the response to insonifications.
- Avoid the use of cosmetic filters and specific imaging modalities such as Harmonic Imaging, Contrast, Doppler, Compounding.
- Achieve the highest frame rate possible (e.g., no persistence, no multifocusing).
- Save the data in DICOM format. In case, this is not possible, save the data directly as a video format. Visual findings, especially when related to very small alterations, do not appear on every frame. It is thus advantageous to acquire movies, where the lung surface below the landmark can be monitored for few seconds during breathing.

5.5 Lung Ultrasonography Findings

The typical LUS pattern of COVID-19 pneumonia is the patchy and bilateral distribution of the main lesions [30, 43]. Typical LUS findings can be found in all lung fields, although bilateral posterior/lateral ones are more frequently involved [30, 44].

In general, the basic LUS semeiotics of COVID-19 pneumonia does not differs in adults and children, with the pleural line irregularities, vertical artifacts, white lung and subpleural consolidations being the main described findings. However, most of these patterns are less frequently seen in children than adults, probably because severe forms of COVID-19 pneumonia are less common in this age group. Therefore, although described, wide and diffuse areas of subpleural consolidations are rare, while in children are more frequently seen diffuse short and long artifacts and isolated small subpleural consolidations. If large consolidations with air bronchogram are seen, bacterial superinfections should be suspected and treated accordingly.

The details of the main LUS patterns are as follow:

- *Pleural line irregularities*, such as thickening or interruptions, caused by the replacement of air with blood, pus, fibrin, according to Huang [30, 44] (Fig. 5.3).
- *B-lines*: vertical artifacts generated by the variation of the acoustic impedance due to the inflammatory process; typically, vertical artifacts in COVID-19 patients are long, touch the bottom of the ultrasound screen, are bright and thick [30] (Figs 5.3 and 5.4).
- *Patchy areas of white lung*: regions of white areas with the absence of A-lines (horizontal and hyperechoic lines due to the normal reflection of the ultrasound beam) and vertical artifacts, that correspond to increased density of the lung parenchyma [30] (Fig. 5.5).
- *Subpleural consolidations*: irregular hypoechoic areas, indicating a collapsed lung or atelectasis [30] (Fig. 5.5).
- *Air bronchograms* and *pleural effusions*: are rare and unusual, their presence should first let the clinician thinking other diagnosis or superinfections [24].
- The presence of small *pleural effusions* may be part of the systemic inflammatory picture in children with a Pediatric Inflammatory Multisystem Syndrome (PIMS) temporally associated with SARS-CoV-2 [8, 11] (Fig. 5.6).

LUS findings are related to the extent of lung injury. In the early stages, the lesions described are irregular vertical artifacts (B-lines) with small regions of white lung. In the intermediate stages, these lesions extend over a larger lung surface. In case of respiratory failure, subpleural consolidations are reported in a gravitational position associated with air bronchograms and large regions of white lung. Furthermore, the diagnostic efficacy of LUS is high especially for severe patients [28–30, 46].

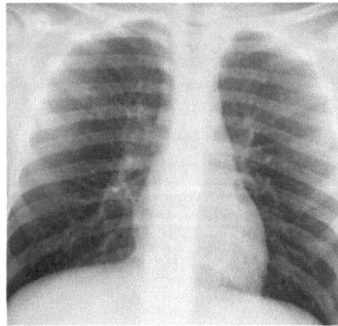 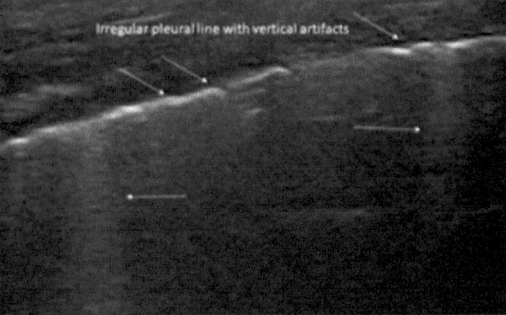

Fig. 5.3 Lung ultrasound findings in a child with COVID-19 pneumonia compared to chest X-ray. LUS shows an irregular pleural line (with thickening and interruptions) and vertical artifacts (*arrows*). The chest X-ray shows a nonspecific picture of slight accentuation of the lung interstitium bilaterally

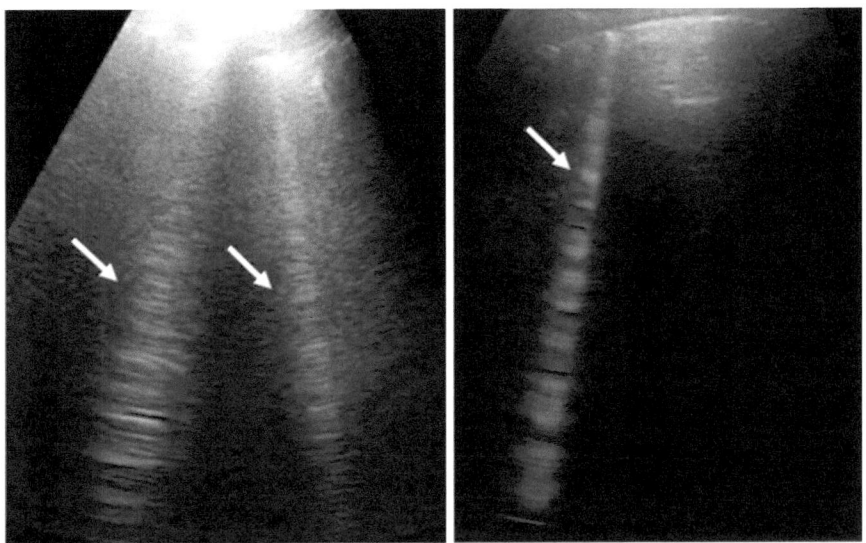

Fig. 5.4 Lung ultrasound findings in a child with COVID-19 pneumonia: patchy areas of bright and thick vertical artifacts (*arrows*)

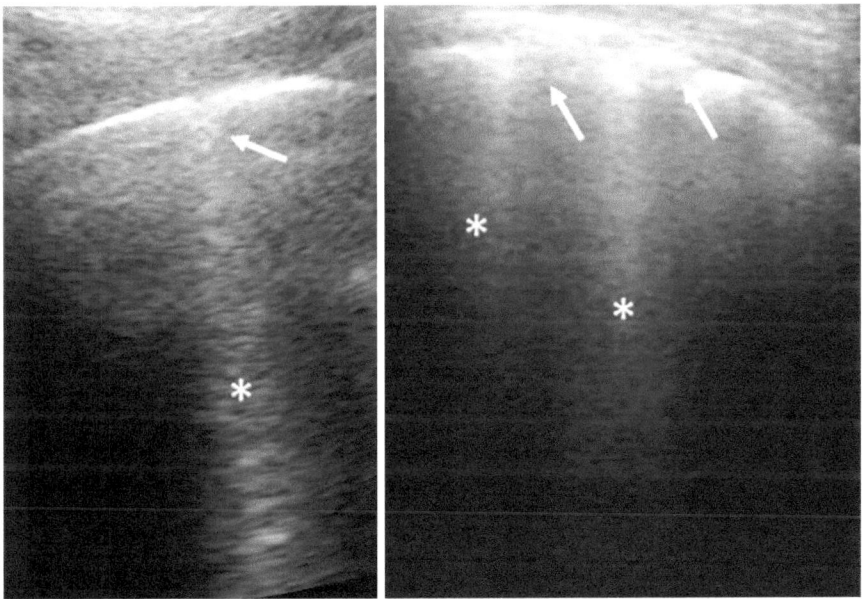

Fig. 5.5 Lung ultrasound findings in child with COVID-19 pneumonia: patchy areas of small subpleural consolidations (hypoechoic areas, *arrows*) and below areas of white lung with multiple, coalescent vertical artifacts (*asterisks*)

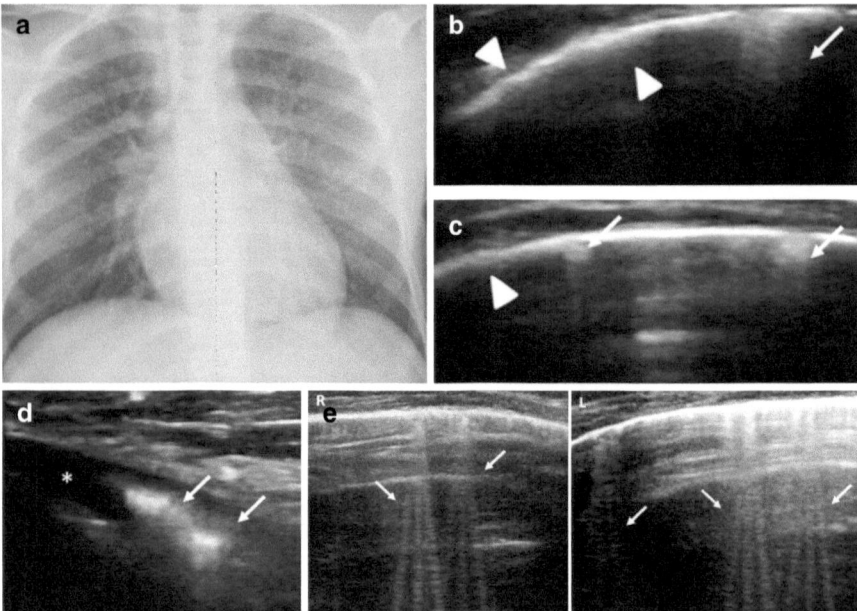

Fig. 5.6 Chest X-ray and lung ultrasound findings in a 10 year old girl with pediatric inflammatory multisystem syndrome temporally associated with SARS-CoV-2 (PIMS-TS). (**a**) The chest X-ray shows a nonspecific picture of accentuation of the lung interstitium bilaterally. (**b, c**) Lung ultrasound shows patchy areas of inflammation characterized by irregularities of the pleural line, which is thickened (*arrowhead*), and short vertical artifacts (*arrow*). (**d**) Lung ultrasound shows a small pleural effusion (*asterisk*) associated to small subpleuric consolidations and below areas of short vertical artifacts (*arrows*). (**e**) Lung ultrasound shows areas of long, basal, bilateral single vertical artifacts (*arrows*) with regular pleural line: picture of interstitial pulmonary edema due to impaired cardiac function caused by the inflammatory systemic process [45]

Consequently, in order to allow comparing the severity of COVID-19 pneumonia of different patients, limiting the subjectivity and the operator dependence of the exam, *Soldati et al.* proposed a *LUS score of severity of COVID-19 related findings* [29]:

- Score 0: normal LUS pattern characterized by regular pleural line and A-lines;
- Score 1: vertical artifacts are described. The pleural line appears indented with several B-lines;
- Score 2: a broken pleural line with dark and white consolidation areas are described;
- Score 3: large regions of white lung.

5.6   PIMS-TS and Point-of-Care Ultrasound

Recently, reports from Europe and North America have described clusters of children and adolescents requiring admission to intensive care units with a multisystem inflammatory condition with some features similar to those of Kawasaki disease and toxic shock syndrome [11, 12]. Case reports and small series have described a presentation of acute illness accompanied by a hyperinflammatory syndrome, leading to multiorgan failure and shock [10]. Initial hypotheses are that this syndrome may be related to COVID-19 based on initial laboratory testing showing positive serology in a majority of patients. Children have been treated with anti-inflammatory treatment, including parenteral immunoglobulin and steroids.

The World Health Organization provided a *preliminary case definition* [11, 12]:

Children and adolescents 0–19 years of age with fever ≥3 days

AND two of the following:

1. Rash or bilateral non-purulent conjunctivitis or muco-cutaneous inflammation signs (oral, hands or feet).
2. Hypotension or shock.
3. Features of myocardial dysfunction, pericarditis, valvulitis, or coronary abnormalities (including ECHO findings or elevated Troponin/NT-proBNP).
4. Evidence of coagulopathy (by PT, PTT, elevated d-Dimers).
5. Acute gastrointestinal problems (diarrhea, vomiting, or abdominal pain).

AND

Elevated markers of inflammation such as ESR, C-reactive protein, or procalcitonin.

AND

No other obvious microbial cause of inflammation, including bacterial sepsis, staphylococcal or streptococcal shock syndromes.

AND

Evidence of COVID-19 (RT-PCR, antigen test or serology positive), or likely contact with patients with COVID-19.

Although the role of Lung Ultrasound has not yet directly evaluated in patients with PIMS-TS, experts in the field and us believe that point-of-care ultrasound (POCUS) can play a primary role in the diagnosis of suspicion and management of children with PIMS-TS. In particular, the following POCUS patterns should be looked for in a child with proven exposure to SARS-CoV-2 virus and signs and symptoms of systemic inflammation (Fig. 5.6):

- Presence of pleural effusions (Fig. 5.6d)
- Presence of long, basal, bilateral vertical artifacts on lung ultrasound (Fig. 5.6e)
- Presence of pericardial effusion

- Reduced or impaired heart contractility
- Free abdominal fluid, with or without thickening of bowel wall thickening

The presence of one or more of these findings in a child with proven or suspect COVID-19 or known exposure to an adult with SARS-CoV-2 infection, should be considered as a red flag and alert the evaluating physician for possible evolution through PIMS-TS and shock.

5.7   Conclusion

The use of LUS during the COVID-19 outbreak in children has several advantages, such as the bedside execution, the need for fewer operators, and the possibility of performing it even at home and thus avoiding hospitalization of patients and over-crowding of the hospital. It is also less expensive (therefore easier to obtain in a developing country) and does not use ionizing radiation. Also, LUS can be used to monitor patients requiring serial examinations, since it is radiation free.

It is important to highlight that CT and LUS are not competitive but rather complementary tools that can be used in different settings to answer different clinical questions. CT scan offers a comprehensive view of the lung and can also help identify complications such as infarction, embolism, emphysema. LUS can be used as a first level exam during the first evaluation in the pediatric emergency department or even at home to distinguish low risk from high-risk patients. In particularly, in children with mild to moderate disease, the proper use of LUS can allow the physician to avoid unnecessary CT examinations. Also, although not yet extensively studied, LUS and whole body point-of-care ultrasound can help in detecting those children at higher risk of developing PIMS-TS.

Since more studies are needed on the role of LUS in children with COVID-19, we strongly support the sharing of information and data on online platforms in order to better understand prognostic information of LUS findings in pediatric COVID-19, as already suggested by the researchers of the Italian Academy of Thoracic Ultrasound (ADET) [29].

Author Contributions DB and CDR contributed to the conception and design of the chapter and wrote the manuscript, collected the data and the articles, read and approved the final version.

Acknowledgments We wish to express our gratitude to the Italian Academy of Thoracic Ultrasound (ADET, Accademia Di Ecografia Toracica) that provided training, knowledge, inspiration, advices and telematics counseling during the COVID-19 pandemic to all Italian clinicians involved in the COVID-19 forefront.

References

1. Zhu N, Zhang D, Wang W, Li X, Yang B, Song J, et al. A novel coronavirus from patients with pneumonia in China, 2019. N Engl J Med. 2020;382(8):727–33. https://doi.org/10.1056/NEJMoa2001017.
2. Dong Y, Mo X, Hu Y, Qi X, Jiang F, Jiang Z, et al. Epidemiology of COVID-19 among children in China. Pediatrics. 2020;145:e20200702. https://doi.org/10.1542/peds.2020-0702.
3. Lu W, Zhang S, Chen B, Chen J, Xian J, Lin Y, et al. A clinical study of noninvasive assessment of lung lesions in patients with coronavirus disease-19 (COVID-19) by bedside ultrasound. Ultraschall Med. 2020;41(3):300–7. https://doi.org/10.1055/a-1154-8795.
4. Qiu H, Wu J, Hong L, Luo Y, Song Q, Chen D. Clinical and epidemiological features of 36 children with coronavirus disease 2019 (COVID-19) in Zhejiang, China: an observational cohort study. Lancet Infect Dis. 2020;20(6):689–96. https://doi.org/10.1016/S1473-3099(20)30198-5.
5. Tagarro A, Epalza C, Santos M, Sanz-Santaeufemia FJ, Otheo E, Moraleda C, et al. Screening and severity of coronavirus disease 2019 (COVID-19) in children in Madrid, Spain. JAMA Pediatr. 2020:e201346. https://doi.org/10.1001/jamapediatrics.2020.1346.
6. Götzinger F, Santiago-García B, Noguera-Julián A, Lanaspa M, Lancella L, Calò Carducci FI, et al. COVID-19 study group. COVID-19 in children and adolescents in Europe: a multinational, multicentre cohort study. Lancet Child Adolesc Health. 2020;4(9):653–61. https://doi.org/10.1016/S2352-4642(20)30177-2.
7. Parri N, Magistà AM, Marchetti F, Cantoni B, Arrighini A, Romanengo M, et al. Characteristic of COVID-19 infection in pediatric patients: early findings from two Italian Pediatric Research Networks. Eur J Pediatr. 2020;179(8):1315–23. https://doi.org/10.1007/s00431-020-03683-8.
8. Riphagen S, Gomez X, Gonzalez-Martinez C, Wilkinson N, Theocharis P. Hyperinflammatory shock in children during COVID-19 pandemic. Lancet. 2020;395(10237):1607–8. https://doi.org/10.1016/S0140-6736(20)31094-1.
9. Paediatric Intensive Care Society (PICS) Statement: increased number of reported cases of novel presentation of multi system inflammatory disease. 2020. https://picsociety.uk/wp-content/uploads/2020/04/PICS-statement-re-novel-KD-C19-presentation-v2-27042020.pdf. Accessed 27 Apr 2020.
10. Health Alert Network (HAN): Multisystem Inflammatory Syndrome in Children (MIS-C) Associated with Coronavirus Disease 2019 (COVID-19). 2020. https://emergency.cdc.gov/han/2020/han00432.asp. Accessed 14 May 2020.
11. European Centre for Disease Prevention and Control Rapid Risk Assessment: paediatric inflammatory multisystem syndrome and SARS-CoV-2 infection in children. 2020. https://www.ecdc.europa.eu/sites/default/files/documents/covid-19-risk-assessment-paediatric-inflammatory-multisystem-syndrome-15-May-2020.pdf. Accessed 15 May 2020.
12. World Health Organization. Scientific Brief: multisystem inflammatory syndrome in children and adolescents with COVID-19. 2020. https://www.who.int/news-room/commentaries/detail/multisystem-inflammatory-syndrome-in-children-and-adolescents-with-covid-19. Accessed 15 May 2020.
13. Licciardi F, Pruccoli G, Denina M, Parodi E, Taglietto M, Rosati S, et al. SARS-CoV-2-induced Kawasaki-like hyperinflammatory syndrome: a novel COVID phenotype in children. Pediatrics. 2020;146(2):e20201711. https://doi.org/10.1542/peds.2020-1711.
14. Verdoni L, Mazza A, Gervasoni A, Martelli L, Ruggeri M, Ciuffreda M, et al. An outbreak of severe Kawasaki-like disease at the Italian epicentre of the SARS-CoV-2 epidemic: an observational cohort study. Lancet. 2020;395:1771. https://doi.org/10.1016/S0140-6736(20)31103-X.
15. Whittaker E, Bamford A, Kenny J, Kaforou M, Jones C, Shah P, et al. Clinical characteristics of 58 children with a pediatric inflammatory multisystem syndrome temporally associated with SARS-CoV-2. JAMA. 2020;8:e2010369. https://doi.org/10.1001/jama.2020.10369.

16. Cheung EW, Zachariah P, Gorelik M, Boneparth A, Kernie SG, Orange JS, et al. Multisystem inflammatory syndrome related to COVID-19 in previously healthy children and adolescents in New York City. JAMA. 2020;8:e2010374. https://doi.org/10.1001/jama.2020.10374.

17. Belhadjer Z, Méot M, Bajolle F, Khraiche D, Legendre A, Abakka S, et al. Acute heart failure in multisystem inflammatory syndrome in children in the context of global SARS-CoV-2 pandemic. Circulation. 2020;142(5):429–36. https://doi.org/10.1161/CIRCULA-TIONAHA.120.048360.

18. Toubiana J, Poirault C, Corsia A, Bajolle F, Fourgeaud J, Angoulvant F, et al. Kawasaki-like multisystem inflammatory syndrome in children during the covid-19 pandemic in Paris, France: prospective observational study. BMJ. 2020;369:m2094. https://doi.org/10.1136/bmj.m2094.

19. Center for Disease Control and Prevention, Center for Preparedness and Response: Multisystem Inflammatory Syndrome in Children (MIS-C) Associated with Coronavirus Disease 2019 (COVID-19), Clinician Outreach and Communication (COCA) Webinar. 2020. https://emergency.cdc.gov/coca/calls/2020/callinfo_051920.asp?deliveryName=USCDC_1052-DM28623. Accessed 19 May 2020.

20. Wang W, Xu Y, Gao R, Lu R, Han K, Wu G, et al. Detection of SARS-CoV-2 in different types of clinical specimens. JAMA. 2020;323(18):1843–4. https://doi.org/10.1001/jama.2020.3786.

21. Ai T, Yang Z, Hou H, Zhan C, Chen C, Lv W, et al. Correlation of chest CT and RT-PCR testing in coronavirus disease 2019 (COVID-19) in China: a report of 1014 cases. Radiology. 2020;26:200642. https://doi.org/10.1148/radiol.2020200642.

22. Rubin GD, Ryerson CJ, Haramati LB, Sverzellati N, Kanne JP, Raoof S, et al. The role of chest imaging in patient management during the COVID-19 pandemic: a multinational consensus statement from the Fleischner society. Radiology. 2020;296(1):172–80. https://doi.org/10.1148/radiol.2020201365.

23. Moro F, Buonsenso D, Moruzzi MC, Inchingolo R, Smargiassi A, Demi L, et al. How to perform lung ultrasound in pregnant women with suspected COVID-19. Ultrasound Obstet Gynecol. 2020;55(5):593–8. https://doi.org/10.1002/uog.22028.

24. Musolino AM, Supino MC, Buonsenso D, Ferro V, Valentini P, Magistrelli A, et al. Lung ultrasound in children with COVID-19: preliminary findings. Ultrasound Med Biol. 2020:S0301-5629(20)30198-8. https://doi.org/10.1016/j.ultrasmedbio.2020.04.026.

25. Buonsenso D, Piano A, Raffaelli F, Bonadia N, de Gaetano DK, Franceschi F. Point-of-care lung ultrasound findings in novel coronavirus disease-19 pneumoniae: a case report and potential applications during COVID-19 outbreak. Eur Rev Med Pharmacol Sci. 2020;24:2776–80. https://doi.org/10.26355/eurrev_202003_20549.

26. Kalafat E, Yaprak E, Cinar G, Varli B, Ozisik S, Uzun C, et al. Lung ultrasound and computed tomographic findings in pregnant woman with COVID-19. Ultrasound Obstet Gynecol. 2020;55(6):835–7. https://doi.org/10.1002/uog.22034.

27. Smith MJ, Hayward SA, Innes SM, Miller A. Point-of-care lung ultrasound in patients with COVID-19 - a narrative review. Anaesthesia. 2020;75(8):1096–104. https://doi.org/10.1111/anae.15082.

28. Peng QY, Wang XT, Zhang LN. Chinese Critical Care Ultrasound Study Group (CCUSG). Findings of lung ultrasonography of novel corona virus pneumonia during the 2019-2020 epidemic. Intensive Care Med. 2020;46(5):849–50. https://doi.org/10.1007/s00134-020-05996-6.

29. Soldati G, Smargiassi A, Inchingolo R, Buonsenso D, Perrone T, Briganti DF, et al. Proposal for international standardization of the use of lung ultrasound for patients with COVID-19: a simple, quantitative, reproducible method. J Ultrasound Med. 2020;39(7):1413–9. https://doi.org/10.1002/jum.15285.

30. Soldati G, Smargiassi A, Inchingolo R, Buonsenso D, Perrone T, Briganti DF, et al. Is there a role for lung ultrasound during the COVID-19 pandemic? J Ultrasound Med. 2020;39(7):1459–62. https://doi.org/10.1002/jum.15284.

31. De Rose C, Inchingolo R, Smargiassi A, Zampino G, Valentini P, Buonsenso D. How to perform pediatric lung ultrasound examinations in the time of COVID-19. J Ultrasound Med. 2020;39(10):2081–2. https://doi.org/10.1002/jum.15306.

32. Parri N, Lenge M, Buonsenso D, Coronavirus Infection in Pediatric Emergency Departments (CONFIDENCE) Research Group. Children with Covid-19 in pediatric emergency departments in Italy. N Engl J Med. 2020;383(2):187–90. https://doi.org/10.1056/NEJMc2007617.
33. Bradley JS, Byington CL, Shah SS, Alverson B, Carter ER, Harrison C, et al. Paediatric Infectious Diseases Society and the Infectious Diseases Society of America. The management of community-acquired pneumonia in infants and children older than 3 months of age: clinical practice guidelines by the Paediatric Infectious Diseases Society and the Infectious Diseases Society of America. Clin Infect Dis. 2011;53:e25–76. https://doi.org/10.1093/cid/cir625.
34. Pereda MA, Chavez MA, Hooper-Miele CC, Gilman RH, Steinhoff MC, Ellington LE, et al. Lung ultrasound for the diagnosis of pneumonia in children: a meta-analysis. Paediatrics. 2015;135:714–22. https://doi.org/10.1542/peds.2014-2833.
35. Berce V, Tomazin M, Gorenjak M, Berce T, Lovren B. The usefulness of lung ultrasound for the aetiological diagnosis of community-acquired pneumonia in children. Sci Rep. 2019;9(1):17957. https://doi.org/10.1038/s41598-019-54499-y.
36. Musolino AM, Tomà P, Supino MC, Scialanga B, Mesturino A, Scateni S, et al. Lung ultrasound features of children with complicated and non-complicated community acquired pneumonia: a prospective study. Pediatr Pulmonol. 2019;54:1479–86. https://doi.org/10.1002/ppul.24426.
37. Supino MC, Buonsenso D, Scateni S, Scialanga B, Mesturino MA, Bock C, et al. Point-of-care lung ultrasound in infants with bronchiolitis in the paediatric emergency department: a prospective study. Eur J Pediatr. 2019;178:623–32. https://doi.org/10.1007/s00431-019-03335-6.
38. Buonsenso D, Brancato F, Valentini P, Curatola A, Supino M, Musolino AM. The use of lung ultrasound to monitor the antibiotic response of community-acquired pneumonia in children: a preliminary hypothesis. J Ultrasound Med. 2020;39:817–26. https://doi.org/10.1002/jum.15147.
39. Copetti R. Is lung ultrasound the stethoscope of the new millennium? Definitely yes! Acta Med Acad. 2016;45:80–1. https://doi.org/10.5644/ama2006-124.162.
40. Buonsenso D, Pata D, Chiaretti A. COVID-19 outbreak: less stethoscope, more ultrasound. Lancet Respir Med. 2020;8(5):e27. https://doi.org/10.1016/S2213-2600(20)30120-X.
41. Kampf G, Todt D, Pfaender S, Steinmann E. Persistence of coronaviruses on inanimate surfaces and their inactivation with biocidal agents. J Hosp Infect. 2020;104(3):246251. https://doi.org/10.1016/j.jhin.2020.01.022.
42. World Health Organization. Medical devices: personal protective equipment. In: World Health Organization website. 2020. https://www.who.int/medical_devices/meddev_ppe/en/. Accessed 6 Mar 2020.
43. Volpicelli G, Gargani L. Sonographic signs and patterns of COVID-19 pneumonia. Ultrasound J. 2020;12(1):22. https://doi.org/10.1186/s13089-020-00171-w.
44. Huang Y, Wang S, Liu Y, Zhang Y, Zheng C, Zheng Y, et al. A preliminary study on the ultrasonic manifestations of peripulmonary lesions of non-critical novel coronavirus pneumonia (COVID-19). Available at SSRN. 2020. https://doi.org/10.21203/rs.2.24369/v1.
45. Kirchhoff C, Leidel BA, Kirchhoff S, Braunstein V, Bogner V, Kreimeier U, et al. Analysis of N-terminal pro-B-type natriuretic peptide and cardiac index in multiple injured patients: a prospective cohort study. Crit Care. 2008;12(5):R118. https://doi.org/10.1186/cc7013.
46. Poggiali E, Dacrema A, Bastoni D, Tinelli V, Demichele E, Ramos PM, et al. Can lung US help critical care clinicians in the early diagnosis of novel coronavirus (COVID-19) pneumonia? Radiology. 2020;295(3):E6. https://doi.org/10.1148/radiol.2020200847.

Lennard M. Gettz and Robert L. Bard

6.1 Introduction

In April of 2020, a collaborative research project to explore (and design) a working model for remote ultrasound training and diagnostic evaluation was formed with the hopes of formalizing a future strategy of "virtualizing" technology-based health assessments. Code named "SalScan," this concept was formulated between a research strategist & process analyst, a NYC based radiologist, a volunteer patient who tested Covid negative, a portable ultrasound manufacturer (who donated their latest portable ultrasound model), and a remote/virtual training specialist to conduct imaging guidance to ensure the patient's proper use of the device. The developers hoped to formalize this protocol as a nationwide scanning alternative during Covid times, as it was first launched in European triage centers to identify covid-related respiratory disorders [1] (Figs. 6.1 and 6.2).

The SalScan test program was established to review, record, and build conclusive evidence of any/all useful information that may lead to, or reflect the strategic paradigms of real-life applications pertaining to the use of remote personal and portable ultrasound.

Supplementary Information The online version of this chapter (https://doi.org/10.1007/978-3-030-66614-9_6) contains supplementary material, which is available to authorized users.

L. M. Gettz (✉)
NY Cancer Resource Alliance, New York, NY, USA
e-mail: lg@321image.com

R. L. Bard
Bard Cancer Center, New York, NY, USA
e-mail: rbard@cancerscan.com

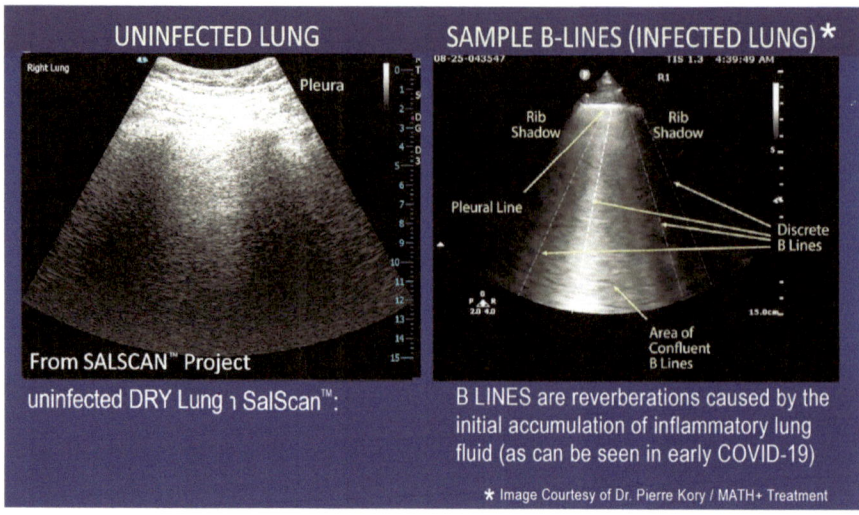

Fig. 6.1 Normal lung scan (left) abnormal lung with B-lines (right)

Fig. 6.2 Positive test for COVID image courtesy of patient

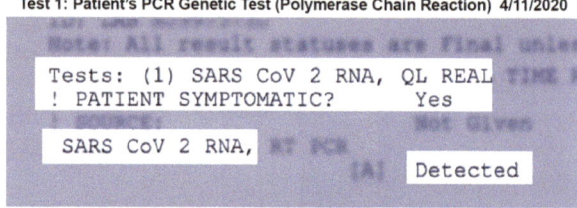

6.2   Testing Parameters

Objectives of the SalScan test program include (Fig. 6.3):

1. Creating a synergistic work model of the three integral participants (the patient, the trainer and the overreader/radiologist) to support a future work plan for any and all remote diagnostic scenarios
2. Blueprinting and monitoring the progress of a working model of a medically monitored self-scanning paradigm (including scan diagrams on the torso, selected probes and frequency settings)
3. Developing any and all instructional guidelines to duplicate the process of this plan

4. Selecting and reviewing portable ultrasound technology with easy-to-use controls for ANY patient
5. Tracking the feasibility of a patient-induced tele-training program to capture ultrasound images for medical diagnosis via telemedicine
6. Challenging the current web-based communication solutions, including conferencing, file sharing, privacy protocols, media player applications, and collaboration (group) reporting capabilities
7. Developing a fully functioning remote training program (through the use of web-based teleconferencing) to guide the patient on the proper/effective use of ultrasound transducers or probes
8. Assessing the actual "learning curve" of the patient to confirm a formatted lesson plan
9. Evaluating the UI (user interface) of the current technology controls to identify patient's learning success
10. Reviewing, overcoming and problem-solving all obstacles of the remote connection
11. Develop a fully streamlined data transferring/file sharing portal with the over-reader (radiologist) to assess and submit a full report of the patient's condition
12. Producing a quantitative data-gathering screening program from a home-based unit
13. Exploring and confirming the effectiveness of a portable ultrasound as a screening option for any field (non-hospital) situation—i.e., battlefields, the ER, ocean liners, ambulances, space programs, natural disasters, etc.
14. Promoting a safety-conscious program to test for contagious pathogens in the safely and comforts of one's own home without health risks from travel
15. Developing a solid 3-point communication system for a real-time remote diagnostic protocol; synergy between patient, trainer and radiologist
16. Opening many more potential patient types, disorders and scenarios for this level of remote scanning access and telemedicine

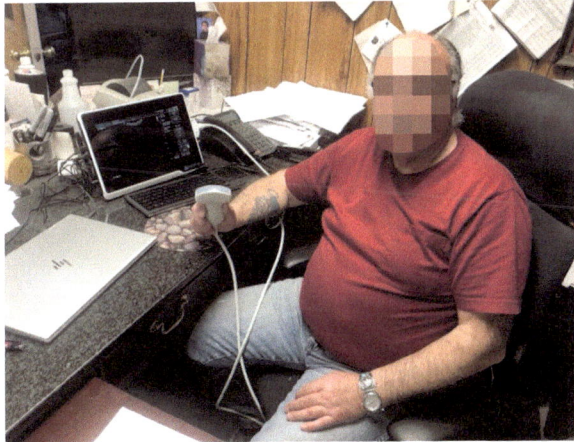

Fig. 6.3 Picture of patient using portable home unit image courtesy of patient

This self-screening program is an opportunity to beta-test key elements of the remote instructional functions and medical diagnostic intervention whereby the project planner can successfully track and explore all procedural responses and the many findings set by the dynamics between the three parties: *the patient, the radiologist, and the remote trainer.*

The obstacles of zero physical contact and the scenario of conducting a scan training to the a nonmedically familiar individual aimed to draw valuable conclusions dedicated to reproducing this remote screening plan for countless emergency and nonurgent care situations worldwide.

The volunteer patient (Mr. Sal Banchitta) offered his own Covid-test results, his experiences and his complete participation to this technical process research. The program directors were successfully able to conduct a real-time beta-test that drafts a complete staging plan on a future of remote virtual ultrasound screening.

6.3   Advancing the Remote Scan Movement and Pre-hospital Ultrasound

Before Covid-19, TeleMedicine, TeleHospital, and other web-based "tech med" solutions have existed for decades. Teleradiology has been used for over 60 years since film was being passed through a digitizer for direct digital capturing and transmitting globally overnight [2]. This allowed faster response when it comes to head injuries in rural areas and other trauma events where teleradiology vastly improved other applications in diagnosis and treatment planning. Today, expanded evidence of remote imaging appear in areas like space travel, emergency response, military deployments, and pandemics.

Pre-hospital ultrasound has many clinical applications that may reduce morbidity and potentially improve outcomes for patients with life-threating conditions. Remote ultrasound telemedical services were developed nationally by the author (Dr Bard) in 1980 and military field hospital application by Dr. Ted Harcke for the US Armed Services in the in the 1990s for imaged guided removal of foreign bodies. Worldwide, responders have adopted the use of a portable noninvasive, nonradiation ultrasound in their rescue rig. For example, in Germany, the use of ultrasound in the field has focused on the FAST exam and cardiac sonography for nontraumatic patients since 2002–2003. French prehospital clinicians have adopted ultrasound in certain areas as well, including SAMU (Service d'Aide Médicale d'Urgence). The Italian EMS system began incorporating ultrasound into prehospital care in 2005 [3].

Prehospital ultrasound is employed in this setting to differentiate reversible causes of pulseless electrical activity (PEA), assess for pericardial, intraperitoneal, and pleural fluid in trauma, and to differentiate between pulmonary edema and emphysema. In the USA, the focus on rapid transport and limiting on-scene time may have contributed to slower adoption of prehospital ultrasound [3].

6.4 Initializing the Remote Self-Screening Concept and Process

The patient volunteered himself to be the first test case and self-scanning trainee for a regimen of chest ultrasound scans under the beta-tested REMOTE HOME-SCAN AND TELE-RADIOLOGY program. This program adapted key elements of lung ultrasound for a wider set of uses at the safety and comfort of the patient's home for regular ultrasound screening and continued monitoring.

Targets Provide the patient and overreader and designated radiologist immediate access to a reliable high-frequency PORTABLE ultrasound scans of LUNGS, HEART, LIVER and KIDNEYS (image-R)—the major organs that may show signs of Covid related disorders.

Predictions Imaging results are collected from the test subject (Sal) who is assigned to scan himself regularly within a given window of time (6 consecutive days). In this case, Sal happens to be Covid + but has been recorded to NOT show symptoms. Use of the ultrasound can either confirm that he is in fact asymptomatic, or may identify any hidden anomalies.

Virtual (Web) Access Through complete remote access, the professional ultrasound trainer (Mike Thury) operates the scanning software (via Teamviewer™) while instructing the patient via video conferencing (Zoom™) on how to properly operate the hand held probes and the ultrasound.

Data Collection Routine After each scanning session, the patient and trainer shall save all daily scan images collected—both on the portable device and on a cloud-based backup. Once the given number of days have been satisfied, the designated medical radiologist (Dr. Robert L. Bard, NYC) shall access the device to collect & review all image files for a thorough analysis.

Communication Between the Three Parties (Image-L) Through the use of TeleMedicine and online access of the device's controls and its saved files, the patient has unlimited personal use of a high-frequency portable ultrasound while being remotely guided by a certified ultrasound instructor to scan specific organs of concern. The remote Chest Ultrasound test puts the patient in the driver's seat to safely monitor and receive diagnoses of their own condition.

6.5   Remote Ultrasound Benefits for All Patient Types

The constant evolution and upgrades in portable ultrasound innovations has made it possible for any patient undergoing treatment to track their own progress on a regular schedule (from home) without the hindrance of traveling to a doctor's office. For patients suffering chronic conditions, personal access to a portable ultrasound with remote access to a designated clinical team represents the next generation of patient diagnostic care [4].

During his training and scanning period, the patient's participation provided the SalScan program with important procedural data toward the foundation for this upcoming national screening initiative. Our program developers' goals aim to support the global use of ultrasound imaging devices for the many nonhospital applications where access to large-format devices are simply not available. Use of the ultrasound can either confirm the patient is in fact asymptomatic, or may prove to be useful as an early detection device by identifying any hidden anomalies.

Covid-19 is a multifocal, multiorgan disease meaning that a unit would require variable probes and equipment settings. The settings used in this scan series that included the lungs, liver, kidneys, and heart utilized safety protocols for mechanical index (MI) and thermal index (TIS) employing curved array probe for lung, liver and kidneys and sector scanner for heart and lungs. Different transducers are available on many units but this study did not involve the application of the linear probe since the regions insonated were appropriately covered by the sector and curved array, or linear transducer if necessary.

6.5.1   MI: The Mechanical Index

MI is of possible clinical interest if the beam focus is close to the surface of lung tissue.

MI has the following characteristics:

- *Potential bioeffect*: Any possible mechanical or nonthermal mechanisms—although the likelihood of adverse consequences from these causes is not well understood, such risk may be highest in the presence of gas-saturated structures such as lung tissue.
- *Mode type*: Calculated for all modes of operation.
- *Tissue type and location*: Soft tissue at all locations in the scan field.
- *Acoustic parameter*: Maximum negative (rarefactional) ultrasound pressure at focus.

6.5.2   TIS: The Soft-Tissue Thermal Index

TIS is of interest in the absence of bone, either at the tissue surface or near the beam focus. Applications of clinical interest include general abdominal examinations, first-trimester scanning before fetal bone has ossified, and cardiology. TIS has the following characteristics.

- *Potential bioeffect*: Thermal heating of soft tissue due to absorption of ultrasound. The TIS value is the ratio of the current probe power to the reference level that would cause a 1 °C temperature rise in soft tissue.
- *Mode type*: Relevant for all modes, in both scanned and non-scanned modes.
- *Tissue type and location*: In scanned modes, soft tissue at the surface is of concern. In non-scanned modes, heating of soft tissue along the beam axis between the surface and focus is considered.
- *Acoustic parameters*: For scanned modes, the associated intensity at the surface is usually related to surface tissue heating. For unscanned modes, the maximum derated power through a 1 cm^2 area anywhere along the beam axis is the basis for estimating tissue heating: unscanned beams less than 1 cm^2 in area at the surface are assumed to contribute only to surface heating, and the calculated effects are combined with those of scanned modes to estimate total soft-tissue heating at the surface. Unscanned beams larger than 1 cm^2 at the surface are assumed to heat tissue only near the focus. Total heating effects at the surface and focus are compiled separately, and the larger value is reported as TIS.

The role of the patient includes turning on the unit and applying gel to the areas to be scanned. Wifi internet is activated for real-time connectivity. The sonogram unit activated by the patient will then be used by the remote trainer through video or audio/video conferencing to guide the procedure.

The role of the remote trainer/technician is to view the probe position on the patient and adjust the perpendicularity of the sound beam on the televised image. Breathing and other respiratory maneuvers may be adjusted at this time such as investigation of the inferior vena cava when pericardial effusion is discovered or aberrant ventricular wall motion is present. All imaging functions of the probe such as patient ID input, M mode, Doppler, video are remotely carried out by the trainer during the live scanning session. Routinely, 2–5 s videos are recorded for review and verification of the event.

The role of the physician radiologist is to verify the image quality, probe placement, depth of penetration, and confer with the trainer if adjustments are necessary. Ideally, this interaction occurs at the initial or second visit. Most patients will have normal findings therefore 12 h intervals is adequate for observation. Any aggravation of the symptoms (dypnea, palpitation, oxygen concentration decrease) calls for 4-h scan intervals and real-time physician input. Adverse outcomes may occur at any time and in any organ system. It is recommended that the heart, liver and renal structures be interrogated daily as well since delayed onset of ventricular inflammation (myositis) or large vessel thromboembolic phenomena are increasingly common. If neurologic sequelae occur, the linear probe may image the carotid artery in the neck and the ophthalmic artery/vein complex. The sector or phased array cardiac probe has sufficient penetration to assess the intracranial arteries (transcranial Doppler ultrasound) and check for impending stroke or venous thrombosis.

Overall pulmonary function clinical assessment relates to the A-lines and B-lines. The high percentage of normal pleural A-line appearance implies that there is no significant pleuro-pulmonary pathology as is expected in patients on bedrest. B-line increase may call for hospitalization while the conversion of B-lines to A-lines highlights improvement. Bedside point of care remote diagnostic criteria are not available for non-pulmonary organs. In the "Salscan" project A-line pattern was uniform for 14 days and our patient returned to normal activity. He is currently donating his plasma for the benefit of others.

6.6   Remote CT and Sonogram Fusion Diagnostics

After initial experience with the outpatient remote ultrasound program, the scope moved to remote CT reviews and finally, combined reporting of lung ultrasound with lung CT with the option of image-guided treatment using fusion of both modalities (fusion is covered in chapters 3 and 8) at distant locations throughout the United State on inpatients. On one encounter during the month of June, remote CT review by a radiologist supported the clinical impressions by overworked clinical colleagues. Below are the pertinent data.

6.6.1   Data

6/24/20	CT Initial film	Follow up
Thickened pleura	5/5	1/5
Ground glass opacity (GGO)	5/5	2/5
Subpleural consolidaton	5/5	1/5
Translobar consolidation	5/5	0/5
Multilobar consolidation	5/5	0/5
Pleural effusion	N/A	0/5

6.7   Salscan Project: Statement of Conclusion

1. The SalScan Remote Screening project started on April 15, 2020 for six (6) consecutive days. It collected complete ultrasound video images of the patient's lungs (from various angles), heart, liver, and kidneys each day.
2. As of June 1, 2020, the SalScan project concluded its imaging, multi-testing and research efforts showing a non-symptomatic Covid Positive case. This supports conclusive data available in current medical reports from nationwide testing.
3. The SalScan project integrated the results of the patient's (1) original Covid test and (2) an independent Antibody test.
   (a) The Covid Positive test result assumed the connection with the patient's heavy Flu-like and respiratory symptoms in early January–Feb. and may have functionally recovered by April as our imaging scans have indicated no present physical traces of pathogen response in the major organs scanned.

(b) The patient's recent antibody test indicated positive (+) results, suggesting the validity of the initial Covid test and its diagnostic result. Based on current scientific reports, this presence of antibodies suggest a likelihood of infection by Covid-19 pathogens in the recent past and that the patient's immune system has built up a protein defense to fight the virus.

(c) Our 6-day scan series recognizes his path to recovery (from his noted symptoms from earlier months) as images gathered on April, 2020 have concluded NO visual trace of pathogen response or infections.

4. The SalScan Program was designed as a PILOT to beta-test the blueprint of future Chest Ultrasound Screening, Remote Personal Screening and Virtual Overreading programs.

5. The SalScan Pilot successfully supported the comprehensive breakdown of the 3-member virtual/remote diagnostic paradigm, whereby this test proves the ease of use of the device and its comprehensive application of web-based communication and file sharing technology.

6. As the SalScan volunteer patient continued to maintain a non-symptomatic state (after July) under a twice confirmed Covid Positive test diagnoses, initiating the use of a personal ultrasound screening helped validate the patient's recovery and/ or noncritical status. This also provided necessary peace of mind to the patient seeking to affirm the direction of his clinical test results.

7. Additional imaging studies, medical (lab) reports and peer-reviewed data shall continue on a quarterly basis due to any possible recurrence that may arise. Probability of recurrence has been clearly documented in recent medical journals and news reports.

8. The current pandemic and the growing list of treatment communities are poised to receive this report as part of Dr. Robert Bard's global advocacy to expand the medical use of portable ultrasound in "the front lines" of health responders community.

9. The SalScan virtual remote self-screening protocol, its staging plans, chest ultrasound mapping, scheduling and training process is a comprehensive program design that can be translated to serve any individual undergoing critical care, patients who are recovering from treatments at home or are in remote areas where regular radiology visits may prove to be a hardship to the patient.

Special thanks to Terason Ultrasound for helping to make this project a reality.

CHEST ULTRASOUND SCANNING MAP & PROBE ANGLE

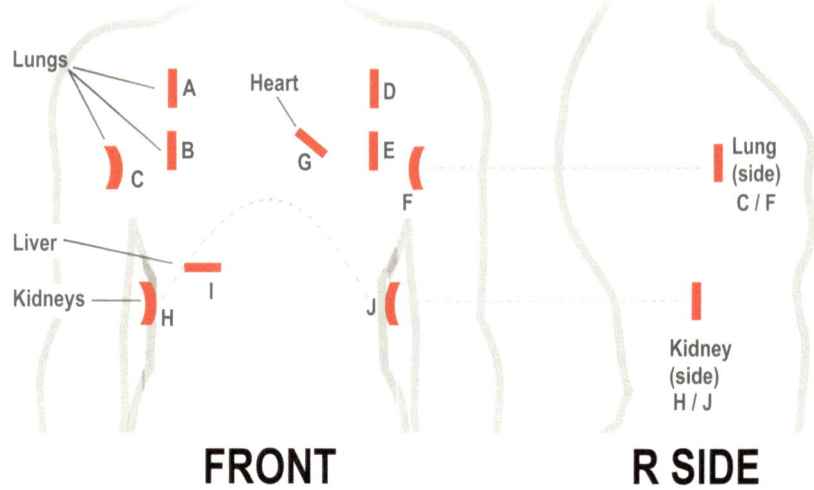

Fig. 6.4 Diagram of probe positions for scan copyright intermediaworx

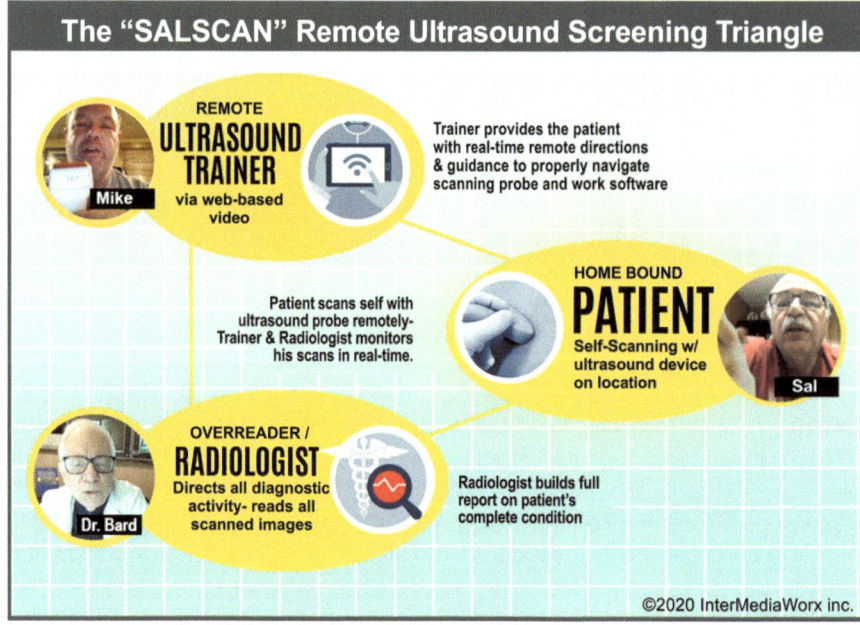

Fig. 6.5 Diagram of roles of radiologist, patient and remote trainer

References

1. Global medical allies share lung ultrasound solution for COVID-19 triage. ITN Imaging Technology news. Apr 6, 2020. https://www.itnonline.com/content/global-medical-allies-share-lung-ultrasound-solution-covid-19-triage. Accessed 2 May 2020.
2. The evolution of telehealth: where have we been and where are we going? https://www.ncbi.nlm.nih.gov/books/NBK207141/. Copyright 2012 by the National Academy of Sciences. All rights reserved. Accessed 1 May 2020.
3. Use of ultrasound by emergency medical services: a review. US Natl. Library of Medicine (PMC); Nov 2011. https://www.ncbi.nlm.nih.gov/pmc/articles/PMC2657261/. Accessed 1 May 2020.
4. Recent developments in tele-ultrasonography. US Natl. Library of Medicine (PMC); Apr–Jun 2018. https://www.ncbi.nlm.nih.gov/pmc/articles/PMC6320468/. Accessed 1 May 2020.

COVID-19 3D/4D Doppler Imaging

Robert L. Bard

7.1 Introduction

In addition to the sonographic characteristics of the B-mode image, the type of vascularization is important for clinical assessment of a lesion in terms of differential diagnosis. In sonographic examinations, the established procedures of power or color-Doppler sonography and contrast enhanced ultrasonography (CEUS) are used for this purpose. Recently color-Doppler sonography characteristics of bacterial pneumonia, obstructive atelectasis, lung infiltrates and bronchial carcinoma have been described. Preliminary studies show that CEUS can be performed on the chest. Various diseases of the lung are characterized by specific contrast sonography findings. The purpose is to describe color/power Doppler sonography and CEUS findings in the presence of peripheral lung consolidations.

7.2 Pathophysiology

The lung is characterized by dual vascularization. Perfusion is achieved on the one hand by lung circulation responsible for pulmonary gas exchange. Lung circulation is accomplished by the pulmonary arteries and their ramifications as well as venules and lung veins. The lung itself is nourished by the bronchial arteries. In contrast to systemic circulation, circulation by the pulmonary arteries is characterized by elastic arteries and their initial branches. The downstream arteries have inelastic muscular walls and from the arterioles onward are partly muscular precapillaries. In contrast to systemic circulation in which arterioles are the main vessels of resistance, in lung circulation the resistance is equally distributed between arteries,

R. L. Bard (✉)
Bard Diagnostics, New York, NY, USA
e-mail: rbard@cancerscan.com

capillaries and veins. Flow in the pulmonary arteries and capillaries is pulsatile and not continuous. In contrast to hypoxic vasodilatation in the systemic circulation, hypoxic vasoconstriction occurs in lung circulation. When lung tissue is affected by a malignant tumor, the carcinoma invades the pulmonary arteries of the affected lung segment where the center of the tumor shows irregular and tortuous vascular patterns. Vascularization is reduced by stenosis, shunting, arteriovenous fistulae, and occlusion of the pulmonary arteries. The bronchial arteries originate on the left side from the aortic arch and on the right side from the intercostal artery forming a vascular ring at the hilum of the lung. Anastomoses between the two systems that are normally closed become open owing to hypoxia and blood supply is provided by bronchial arteries. Angiographic studies show peripheral lung diseases at the pleural wall, such as benign cavitary lesions, lung cysts, lung abscesses and liquefying pneumonia, are nourished by bronchial arteries [1]. However, malignant primary lung tumors and lung metastases are vascularized by bronchial arteries. The intercostal arteries originate from the thoracic aorta and run a strictly intercostal course in the chest wall along the ribs. They are the only vessels visualized on sonography, even in healthy volunteers. Particularly in cases of lesions in the chest wall, these vessels play an important role in tumor vascularization since neoangiogenesis of primary bronchial carcinomas mainly originates in the bronchial arteries. The use of contrast-assisted sonography allows microvessels whose width is larger than that of capillaries to be visualized [2].

7.3   Vascular Imaging Options

Blood flow evaluation measures inflammatory activity, tumor aggression and locates peripheral vascular disorders providing a map for vessel reconstruction with Doppler analysis. CT and MRI vascular studies are invasive and not readily available in outpatient settings. Blue, white and red digits are commonly reported in Covid-19 patients worldwide and this entity is well imaged by Doppler ultrasound. This process of coagulopathy and pulmonary thromboembolism producing lung infarction appears as an absence of vascularization (Fig. 7.1).

7.3.1   Microvessel Imaging

Doppler flow imaging is not depth limited while the new optical technologies of OCT (optical coherence tomography) and RCM (reflectance confocal microscopy) rule out malignant neovascularity that show surface vessels up to 1.5 mm in tissue depth for OCT (0.3 mm for RCM). These and the latest opticoacoustic technologies will have greater application in the future. Advanced units have B-flow Doppler and capability for contrast enhanced ultrasound (CEUS) technology that may better show the vessels and also the vascular status of the dermis for impending necrosis from hypoxemia. Doppler images of blood flow patterns include disorganized flow (Fig. 7.2), tree shaped vascularization (Fig. 7.3) and arterial turbulences in pneumonia or consolidated areas (Fig. 7.4).

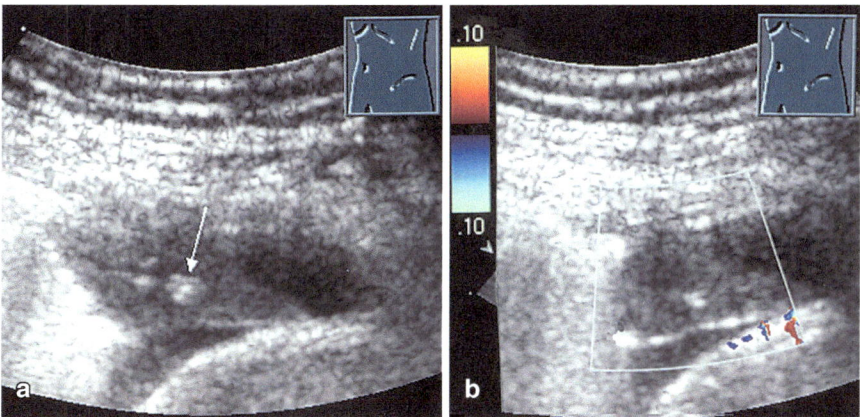

Fig. 7.1 A 43-year-old man with a lung infarction. (**a**) On the B-mode image one finds a hypoechoic wedge-shaped lesion with a central bronchial reflex (*arrow*). (**b**) Color-Doppler sonography shows the absence of vascularization. (THIS FIGURE CORRESPOND TO SPRINGER MATHIS 2O17 LUNG ULTRASOUND CHAPTER 8 with permission)

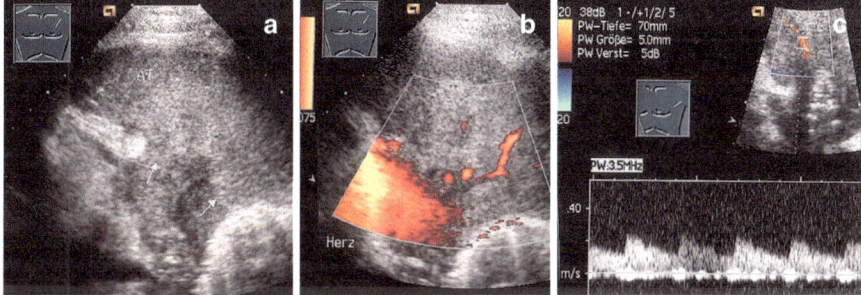

Fig. 7.2 36-year-old man with Hodgkin's disease in the mediastinum. (**a**) On the B-mode image one finds a hypoechoic central tumor formation with atelectasis (*AT*; *arrows*). (**b**) Color-Doppler sonography shows limited vascularization within the atelectasis, which is a sign of constriction of the pulmonary artery. (**c**) Spectral curve analysis shows a monophasic flow signal with reduced arterial flow resistance indicative of bronchial arterial flow. (THIS FIGURE CORRESPOND TO SPRINGER MATHIS 2O17 LUNG ULTRASOUND CHAPTER 8 with permission)

7.3.2   Chest Wall Imaging Limitations

Trauma and iatrogenic chest and breast problems contribute to abnormal chest wall imaging findings on B-mode and Doppler.

Complications are more frequent in patients who have had reconstructive chest or breast surgery or a previous filler (commonly, a nondegradable one), and are injected by a second type of filler, degradable or nondegradable, in the same anatomic region. HA fillers have the very beneficial quality of responding to hyaluronidase, which allows the physician to remove the material. Nevertheless, unwanted side effects with irreversible fillers, are much more difficult to manage, given that total extraction of the filler product may not be possible. Generally, complications

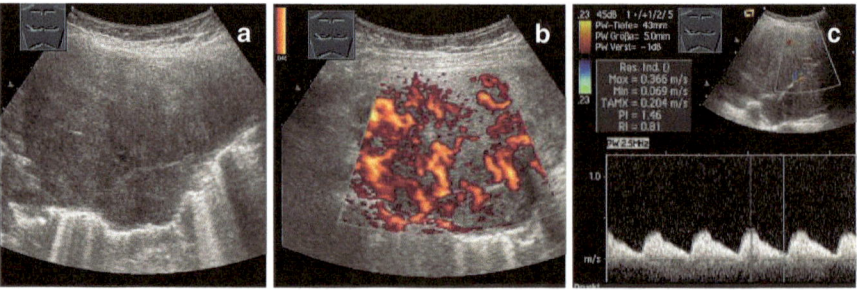

Fig. 7.3 62-year-old man with lung metastases in the presence of renal cell carcinoma. (**a**) The B-mode image reveals a large hypoechoic round lesion. (**b**) Color-Doppler sonography shows strong and disorganized vessels. (**c**) Spectral curve analysis shows a monophasic flow signal indicative of a bronchial artery. (THIS FIGURE CORRESPOND TO SPRINGER MATHIS 2O17 LUNG ULTRASOUND CHAPTER 8 with permission)

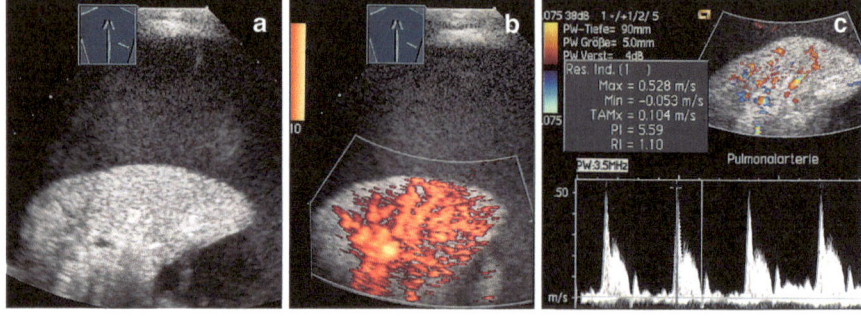

Fig. 7.4 37-year-old man with a pleural effusion and compressive atelectasis. (**a**) The B-mode image reveals a pleural effusion with atelectasis in the lung. (**b**) Color-Doppler sonography shows ramified vascularization. (**c**) Spectral curve analysis shows a high-impedance flow pattern, indicative of a pulmonary artery. (THIS FIGURE CORRESPOND TO SPRINGER MATHIS 2O17 LUNG ULTRASOUND CHAPTER 8 with permission)

are categorized by the onset of adverse event: early events (occurring up to several days post injection) and delayed events (happening from weeks to years post injection). Complications in which ultrasonography plays an important role in diagnosis and management, including dermatopathies, filler migration, hypersensitivity reactions, inflammatory nodules (abscess, granulomas, and panniculitis), noninflammatory nodules (tuberous sclerosis) and vascular complications. Cosmetic material may migrate into areas adjacent to the injection sites, causing swollen areas or palpable masses in the vicinity of injected sites. Furthermore, it is possible to find nondegradable material in local lymph nodes near injected areas, commonly silicone oil which may traverse significant tissue distances.

7.3.3   Vascular Complications

Vascular complications are rare and include injection site necrosis secondary to intravascular injection of filler or external compression of blood supply. Currently, those complications have been mainly reported in literature after HA injections. The most affected arteries are the angular artery of the nasolabial fold and the supratrochlear artery in the glabellar region but intercostal arteries may be affected [3]. Color or power Doppler ultrasound is an important tool in the early detection of vascular obstruction, demonstrating the absence of intraluminal flow, thus confirming the diagnosis or demonstrating area of high velocity due to intrinsic or extrinsic causes. In addition, if the filler injected was HA, ultrasound can guide intravascular hyaluronidase injection, in the exact site of thrombosis, improving the patient's prognosis [4–8].

7.4   Contrast-Assisted Sonography

Similar to power, angio, B-flow or color Doppler sonography, lung infarctions/lung hemorrhages are marked by the absence of contrast enhancement on contrast-assisted sonography. CEUS or contrast-assisted sonography allows the investigator to make a reliable distinction between vascularized and nonvascularized peripheral lung tissue differentiating infarct from compressive atelectasis due to pleural effusion.

7.4.1   Pleurisy

On Color-Doppler Sonography the appearance of pleurisy on the B-mode image is similar to that of a lung infarction. Depending on the size of the invasion, which is transformed into pleural pneumonia, the qualitative color-Doppler sonography characteristically shows pronounced vessels with predominant evidence of an arterial high-impedance flow profile on spectral analysis such as that seen in branches of the pulmonary artery. On Contrast-Assisted Sonography, like color-Doppler sonography findings, pleurisy takes very little time for contrast enhancement to start and is marked by strong contrast enhancement on contrast-assisted sonography. This is indicative of primary vascularization through pulmonary arteries (Fig. 7.5). The value of contrast-assisted sonography lies in its potential for differential diagnosis of nonvascularized peripheral lung lesions such as lung infarction, malignant lesions, or fibrotic scar tissue [9].

7.4.1.1   Color-Doppler Sonography of Focal Round Lesions
A peripheral round lesion of the lung at the wall of the pleura occurring as the cardinal symptom may be due to a benign or malignant lesion. Of decisive importance is the fact that, independent of the cause, the evidence of flow signals is dependent

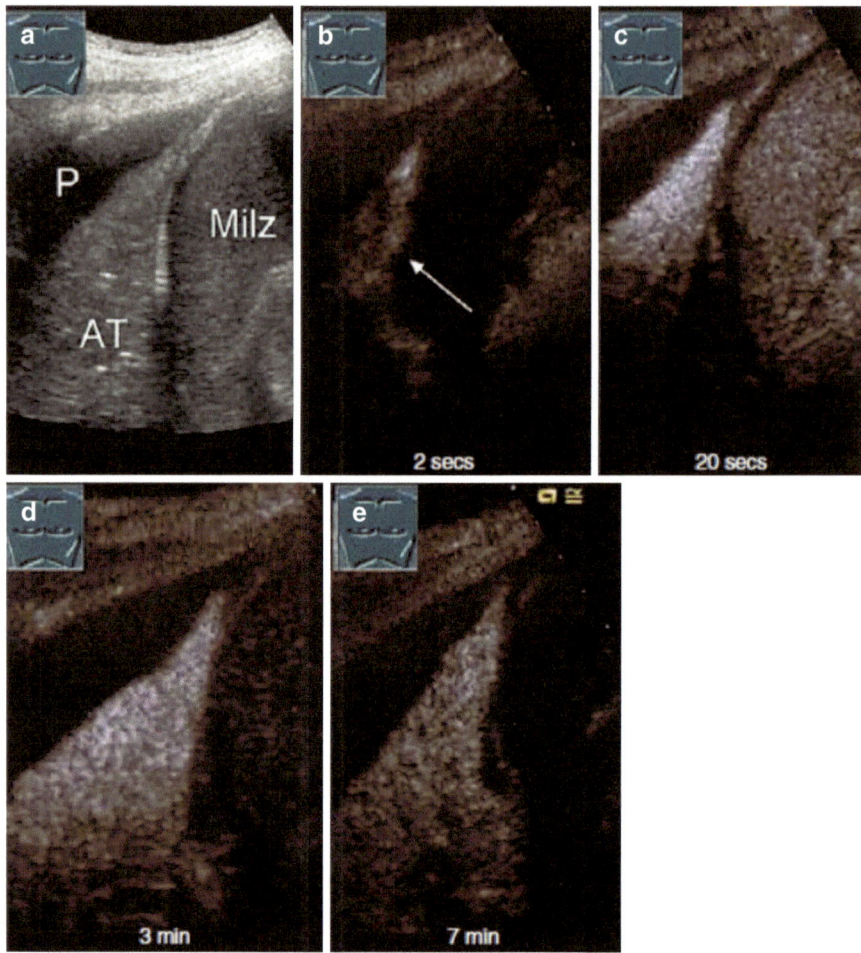

Fig. 7.5 24-year-old man with a pleural effusion and compressive atelectasis in the presence of amyloidosis. (**a**) On the B-mode image one finds a pleural effusion (*P*), an atelectasis (*AT*) and in subcostal location the spleen. Contrast-assisted sonography shows early arterial contrast enhancement after 2 s (**b**). The *arrow* marks the vessel with starting contrast enhancement. After 20 s there is marked contrast enhancement in the atelectatic tissue, which is hyperechoic compared with the parenchyma of the spleen (**c**). In the parenchymatous phase, after 3 min, one finds continued strong contrast enhancement in the atelectasis (**d**), which is also seen after 7 min (**e**). This contrast behavior is indicative of vascularization purely through the pulmonary arteries. (THIS FIGURE CORRESPOND TO SPRINGER MATHIS 2017 LUNG ULTRASOUND CHAPTER 8 with permission)

on the size of the lesion. On careful investigation, one frequently finds arterial high-impedance flow signals from pulmonary arteries and low-impedance flow signals from bronchial arteries in benign as well as malignant peripheral lung lesions. Power or color-Doppler sonography is not currently accepted for distinguishing between benign and malignant peripheral round lesions. In keeping with the variable findings on color-Doppler sonography, contrast-assisted CEUS sonography also shows a heterogeneous pattern of vascularization. Malignant lesions—whether lung metastases or peripheral bronchial carcinomas—are marked by delayed start of contrast enhancement and reduced extent of contrast enhancement indicative of predominant vascularization through bronchial arteries. Depending on the underlying structure, however, lung metastases of renal cell carcinomas, malignant melanoma and frequently, malignant lymphoma show pronounced contrast enhancement, signifying of aggressive tumor angiogenesis. The extent and homogeneity of tumor angiogenesis depend, among other factors, on tumor size. In some cases contrast enhanced ultrasound is useful to assess the malignant or benign nature of the lesion [10].

7.5   Large Lung Consolidation

7.5.1   Pneumonia

7.5.1.1 Color Doppler
Pneumonia is seen on X-rays and sonography in conjunction with the principal finding of a peripheral lung consolidation at the pleural wall. On B-mode image sonography, partial pneumonia demonstrates pronounced air bronchograms while complete consolidation is seen as so-called lung hepatization. On color-Doppler sonography, pneumonia is marked by significantly ramified vessels that correspond to segmental branches of the pulmonary artery. One frequently finds an arterial monophasic flow signal of central bronchial arteries in the invaded lung tissue due to hypoxia. Certain subtypes of adenocarcinoma may appear similar to pneumonia on the B-mode image and on color-Doppler sonography as well. Depending on the extent of hypoxic vasoconstriction in the pulmonary artery, the peripheral vascular tree of pulmonary arteries may not be visualized on qualitative color-Doppler sonography in the presence of advanced pneumonia. Bronchial arteries react to hypoxia by developing vasodilatation, as do all other arteries in the body. This explains the different resistance indices of pneumonia and atelectasis. Thus, in the presence of lobar pneumonia parallel to the pulmonary arteries one occasionally finds an arterial monophasic flow pattern with low resistance indices, indicative of central bronchial arteries. The tuberculous infiltrate is a special phenomenon. It is characterized by marked vessels on color-Doppler sonography in terms of qualitative findings. On spectral analysis, however, it is seen as a monophasic curve, corresponding to bronchial arteries. Cavitary lesions such as tuberculosis, liquefactions, necrosis, abscess, and pseudocysts are characterized by the presence of predominant vascularization through the bronchial artery in the marginal areas around the lesion. Doppler can also be used when evaluating inflammatory or infectious subpleural consolidations, or large consolidations. Presence of flow indicates that something has a better prognosis, that healing can occur because vascularization is present. Lack of color would be a bit more worrisome, as it would mean areas which could be less recoverable. Interest in this area now due to COVID as a means of

assessing an infiltrate as to aggression, and treatment response. Also, the natural course untreated may be followed to resolution by gradual reduction in inflammatory vessels indicated a systemic healing response versus an abrupt loss of neovascularity suggesting infarction [11].

7.5.1.2 Contrast-Assisted Sonography Pneumonia

In keeping with the findings on color-Doppler sonography, classic pneumonia is characterized by a short period until the start of contrast enhancement and strong contrast enhancement on contrast-assisted sonography. This is indicative of predominant vascularization though pulmonary arteries. Reduced contrast enhancement is observed in cases of lobar pneumonia and can be explained by hypoxic vasoconstriction of the pulmonary artery. Delayed contrast enhancement indicates vascularization by the bronchial artery and is observed in cases of liquefaction and chronic pneumonia. Such avascular areas in the region of pneumonia can be clearly demarcated on contrast-assisted sonography. Inhomogeneous contrast enhancement is helpful in identifying typical courses of disease with evidence of consolidation, necrosis, infarct areas, inward bleeding, or abscesses. Especially in parapneumonic echogenic effusions with multiple septa and a suspected pleural empyema, the area can be clearly demarcated from the infiltrated lung [12].

7.5.1.3 Compressive Atelectasis

Color-Doppler Sonography Compressive atelectasis is seen on radiographs and sonography in conjunction with the cardinal finding of a peripheral basal lung consolidation at the pleural wall. The main finding is a pleural effusion, followed by the visualization of compressed lung tissue. On qualitative color-Doppler sonography atelectasis is seen as a strongly ramified vessel. On arterial spectral analysis one usually finds a high-impedance flow signal indicative of pulmonary arteries. Contrast-Assisted Sonography In concurrence with color-Doppler sonography findings, compressive atelectasis is characterized by a brief period until the start of contrast enhancement and strong contrast enhancement on contrast-assisted sonography. This is indicative of vascularization exclusively through the pulmonary arteries. The contrast-assisted sonography pattern of compressive atelectasis is very specific. Round lesions in atelectatic lung tissue are marked by poor contrast enhancement [13].

7.5.1.4 Obstructive Atelectasis

Color-Doppler Sonography The obstructive lung atelectasis is seen as a largely homogeneous hypoechoic transformation on the B-mode image. Depending on the duration of the obstruction, evidence of a "fluid bronchogram" is a characteristic feature in this setting. On qualitative color-Doppler sonography one finds pronounced vessels with evidence of an arterial high-impedance flow signal due to the branches of the pulmonary artery and arterial monophasic flow profile of central bronchial arteries in atelectatic tissue as a result of hypoxia. A frequent finding is the central tumor underlying the atelectasis well imaged since the consolidated atelectatic lung tissue serves as an "acoustic window" to explore central lung structures. This disturbed vascular architecture of the pulmonary artery appears on sonography as reduced or no visualization of vessels in the atelectatic lung tissue. Contrast-Assisted Sonography In keeping with the color-Doppler sonography findings, a recent obstructive atelectasis is marked by the same features as compressive atelectasis—a short period of time until contrast enhancement and strong contrast enhancement on contrast-assisted sonography. This is indicative of atelectatic lung tissue being entirely vascularized by the pulmonary arteries. In this phase, in patients with a central tumor formation, the tumor may be demarcated from atelectatic lung tissue more clearly by contrast-assisted sonography than by B-mode sonography. In cases of obstruction of longer duration, within the atelectasis one may find liquefactions and abscesses. These potential lesions as well as metastases in atelectatic lung tissue can be reliably diagnosed by contrast-assisted sonography. In the course of tumor-related obstructive atelectasis, depending on the structure of the tumor there may be infiltration and occlusion of pulmonary arteries. In this situation contrast-assisted sonography shows delayed start of contrast enhancement and reduced contrast enhancement. This is indicative of a switch to vascularization of atelectatic lung tissue by bronchial arteries. In general the contrast-assisted sonography pattern in cases of obstructive atelectasis is heterogeneous. The pattern of compression atelectasis on contrast enhanced ultrasonography is very specific. In atelectatic lung tissue, round lesions indicative of lung metastases, and wedge-shaped peripheral defects as a sign of infarction, reveal poor or no contrast enhancement. In cases of chronic compression atelectasis, pulmonary artery vascularization may be transformed into purely nutritive bronchial artery vascularization. Contrast enhanced ultrasound can be very valuable in clarifying the etiology of a pleural effusion. An echogenic effusion with multiple septa can be clearly distinguished from tumor tissue and tumor tissue along the pleura from a hematoma or fibrinous tissue [14].

7.5.2 Space-Occupying Lesion of the Chest Wall

7.5.2.1 Color-Doppler Sonography

Sonography is the method of choice to explore the chest wall. The intercostal arteries supplying the chest wall are usually seen even in healthy individuals by the use of color-Doppler sonography. Cystic lesions of the chest wall are usually avascular however a complex and fibrosing mass may envelope the vessels and simulate a solid mass (Fig. 7.6). Fluid filled structures are isodense on conventional chest radiography. Lesions near the heart, mediastinum or great vessels may be interrogated by Doppler before interventions are undertaken (Fig. 7.7). Tumors in the chest wall or pleural metastases are characterized by predominantly intercostal vascularization with a monophasic flow profile when the lesions are adherent to the chest wall. When the tumor has invaded the lung, color-Doppler

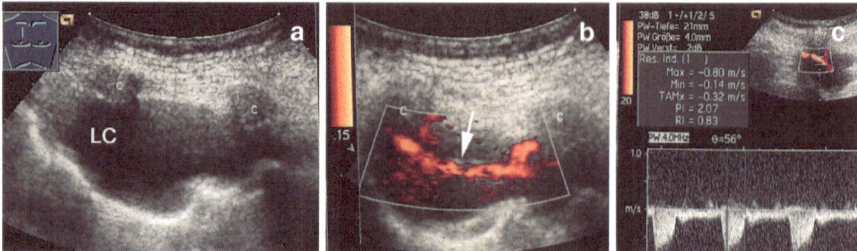

Fig. 7.6 70-year-old man with a primary lung cyst. (**a**) On the B-mode image one finds an anechoic lesion close to the pleura. *C* ribs, *LC* lung cyst. (**b**) Color-Doppler sonography in the power mode shows a strong vessel surrounding the lesion (*arrows*). (**c**) Spectral curve analysis demonstrates a monophasic high-impedance flow signal indicative of an intercostal artery. (THIS FIGURE CORRESPOND TO SPRINGER MATHIS 2017 LUNG ULTRASOUND CHAPTER 8 with permission)

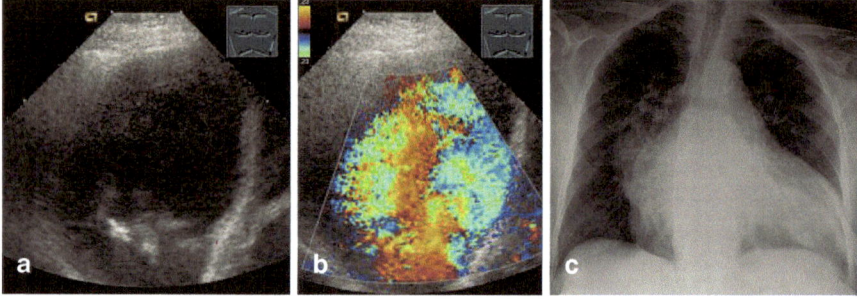

Fig. 7.7 78-year-old woman with dyspnea who came for puncture of a pleural effusion. (**a**) The B-mode image shows an anechoic space-occupying mass in the chest on the left side. (**b**) Color-Doppler sonography reveals a turbulent flow pattern within this lesion, indicative of the left ventricle being located at the chest wall. (**c**) The X-ray shows a large heart; the left ventricle is in contact with the lateral chest wall. (THIS FIGURE CORRESPOND TO SPRINGER MATHIS 2017 LUNG ULTRASOUND CHAPTER 8 with permission)

sonography may show different flow signals as a sign of complex arterial tumor vascularization. The extent of contrast enhancement of the arterial phase may vary. Tumors with pronounced neovascularization reveal strong contrast enhancement. Contrast enhanced ultrasound is very important for the delineation of non-vascularized lesions such as hematomas or abscesses. Solid tumors may have regions of infarcted tissue, fibrosis, immune cell foci or cystic degeneration in any combination. Treatment progress may be misinterpreted if size is used as the sole criteria for efficacy since a certain percentage of malignancies enlarge in size as they are successfully responding. Verification of effect is best ascertained by the use of Doppler or contrast technologies demonstrating quantifiable reduction of feeding vessels (Fig. 7.8) [15].

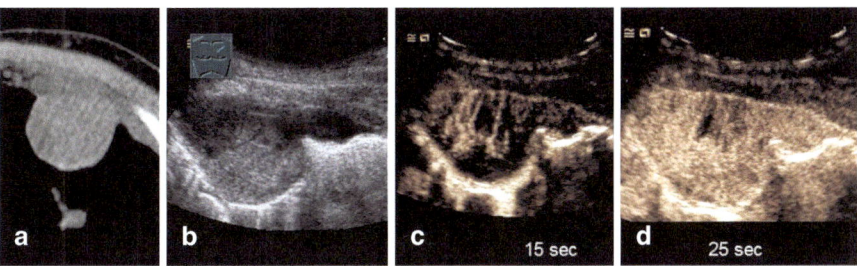

Fig. 7.8 Man with known sarcoma and histologically confirmed multiple lung metastases. (**a**) CT shows a round lesion along the pleura, (**b**) B-mode ultrasound reveals an oval, homogeneous, hypoechoic. Lesion along the pleural margin. (**c**) Contrast-assisted ultrasonography shows, after 15 s, strong enhancement starting from the periphery, as a sign of peripheral vascularization from the bronchial artery. (**d**) After 25 s there is strong and homogeneous contrast enhancement of the lesion, as a sign of marked tumor angiogenesis. (THIS FIGURE CORRESPOND TO SPRINGER MATHIS 2O17 LUNG ULTRASOUND CHAPTER 8 with permission)

7.6 Quantifiable Digital Scanning and Image Guided Interventions

7.6.1 4D Imaging

It is real-time observation of a 3D data set which permits image guided biopsy of the most virulent area of the infiltrate or tumor, targets the densest area of B-Lines or neovascularity and allows the pathologist to focus on the most suspicious region of the lymph node mass excised during surgery. Similarly, during real-time exam the fluid content of a pleural complex cyst maybe aspirated under better visual control and perilesional vessels avoided in a timely manner (Figs. 7.6 and 7.7). This feature enhances the reliability of image-guided treatments and fusion of this data set with CT or MRI scans [16] (Fig. 7.9a–c).

7.6.2 3D/4D Doppler Histogram

In addition to the frequent use of puncture for pleural effusion, space-occupying masses accessible to sonographic investigation, located in the chest wall, pleura, lung or anterior mediastinum, are important indications. Depending on their topographical position and the diagnostic availability and expertise, pathological changes not detectable by a transthoracic approach may be identified diagnostically by one of the interventional procedures displayed in the list in the previous section. Ultrasound assessment of disease activity has been used for adjusting medication dosage so as to follow treatment and not overdose or underdose as necessary in most inflammatory and neoplastic disorders [17].

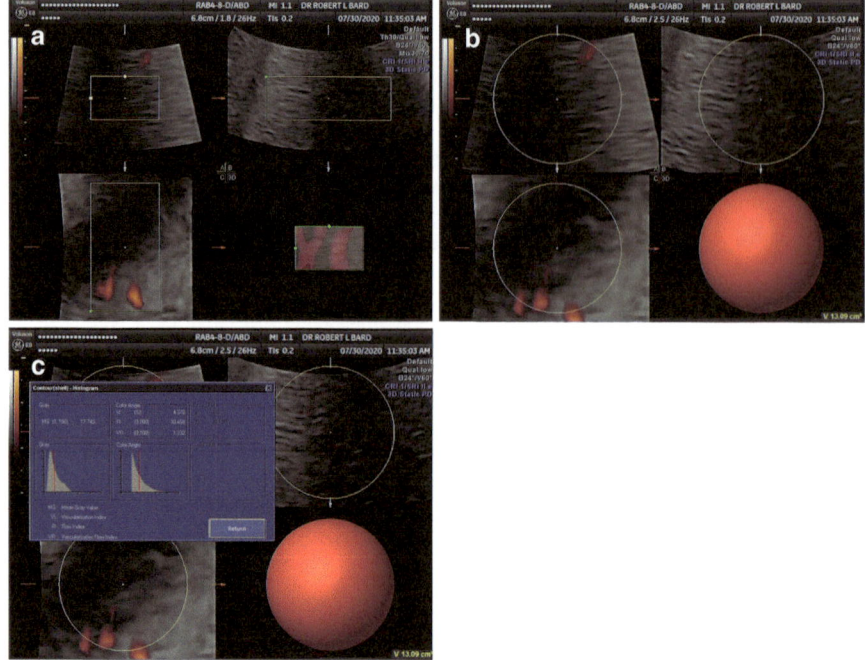

Fig. 7.9 (**a**) 3D multiplanar image of hepatization square show most vascular focus. (**b**) Computer vocal software setup vessel density volumetric. (**c**) 3D Doppler histogram of consolidated lung focus with vessel density (4.37%) which is real time documentation of blood flow that is used as baseline value for follow up. (**a–c Courtesy of Dr Bard**)

7.6.3   Interventions in the Thorax: Indications

1. Space-occupying mass in the thoracic wall (tumors, abscesses, hematomas, changes in the skeletal parts).
2. Space-occupying masses in the pleura.
3. Pleural effusion and pleural empyema (very small quantities, loculated effusions).
4. Peripheral lung consolidations (lung tumor, pneumonia, lung abscess).
5. Mediastinal processes (anterior mediastinum).

Because of the potential risk of complications, the indication for the procedure should be established with care considering the probable comorbidities of the Covid-19 patient. Any sonographically demonstrable space-occupying lesion can be punctured in principle. In a patient who is operable, a suspected malignant tumor located in the periphery will normally not be punctured but will be resected as a first-line measure. Contraindications assuming acceptable coagulation parameters depend on the position of the mass relative to major structures and the invasiveness of the intervention. Urgent interventions require individual assessment of risk. Bullous pulmonary emphysema and pulmonary hypertension are relative contraindications. When respiratory function is severely restricted or blood gas values are poor, a puncture should only be performed when the patient's condition is expected to be improved by the therapeutic intervention. High-risk puncture sites should be avoided. Sonography-guided, CT-guided, or Fusion with CT and MRI are now possible at the bedside with the portable sonographic technologies. The addition of Doppler pre-procedure vessel mapping further reduces blood loss and accidental vascular perforation [3].

7.6.4   3D Lung Doppler

Blood flow is usually measured by 2D Doppler flow with 10% margin of error. 3D volumetric Doppler flows have a 3–5% margin of error and the technology is available on volumetric units. Quantitative blood flow measurements that use pulse wave only are not reliable for use as an imaging biomarker with an accuracy suitable for clinical reliability since it is operator dependent. 3D allows quantitative evaluation of blood flow to end organs to be used as a clinical biomarker [18].

7.7   Summary

Qualitative color-Doppler sonography shows significant findings in certain lung consolidations and is therefore a valuable adjunct to B-mode sonography for etiologic classification of peripheral lung lesions. In keeping with the physiological dual vascularization of the lung by the pulmonary arteries and the bronchial arteries, on color-Doppler sonography one can distinguish between arterial high-impedance spectral curves and arterial low-impedance spectral curves in consolidated lung tissue. Peripheral lung consolidations show characteristic pathologic distribution patterns of pulmonary artery and bronchial artery flow signals that may distinguish malignant from inflammatory processes. Reliable demarcation of vessels of tumor neoangiogenesis is currently not possible with color-Doppler sonography. Experience concerning contrast-assisted sonography in cases of peripheral lung lesions is limited. Contrast-assisted sonography at the chest can be performed easily and rapidly. This modified interventional practice is therefore basically suitable for routine clinical use. Lung lesions can be distinguished by the time they acquire contrast until the start of contrast enhancement and the extent of contrast enhancement. Washout parameters are useful. Initial studies show that contrast-assisted sonography at the chest can be helpful to differentiate ambiguous lung lesions and avoid possible operative complications.

References

1. Mathis G, Dirschmid K. Pulmonary infarctions: sonographic appearance with pathologic correlation. Eur J Radiol. 1993;17:170–4.
2. Mathis G. Chest sonography. Berlin: Springer; 2017.
3. Albrecht T, Blomley M, Bolondi L, et al. Guidelines for the use of contrast agents in ultrasound. Ultraschall Med. 2004;25:249–56.

4. Babo HV, Müller KMG, Huzky A, Bosnjakovic-Buscher S. Die Bronchialarteriographie bei Erkrankungen der Lunge. Radiologe. 1979;19:506–13.
5. Civardi G, Fornari F, Cavanna L, Di Stasi M, Sbolli G, et al. Vascular signals from pleural-based lung lesions studied with pulsed doppler ultrasonography. JCU. 1993;21:617–22.
6. Fissler-Eickhoff A, Müller KM. Pathologie der Pulmonalarterien bei Lungentumoren. DMW. 1994;119:1415–20.
7. Forsberg F, Goldberg BB, Liu BB, et al. Tissue specific US contrast agent for evaluation of hepatic and splenic parenchyma. Radiology. 1999;210:125–32.
8. Bard R. Crescent sign in pulmonary hematoma. USAF J. 1970;2:12–6.
9. Gehmacher O, Kopf A, Scheier M, et al. Can pleurisy be detected with ultrasound? Ultraschall Med. 1997;18:214–9.
10. Gorg C, Seifart U, Holzinger I, et al. Bronchiolo-alveolar carcinoma: sonographic pattern of pneumonia. Eur J Ultrasound. 2002;15:109–17.
11. Gorg C, Seifart U, Gorg K, et al. Color Doppler sonographic mapping of pulmonary lesions: evidence of dual arterial supply by spectral analysis. JUM. 2003;22:1033–9.
12. Gorg C, Bert T. Transcutaneous colour Doppler sonography of lung consolidations: review and pictorial essay. Part 2: colour Doppler sonographic patterns of pulmonary consolidations. Ultraschall Med. 2004;25:285–91.
13. Gorg C, Bert T, Gorg K. Contrast-enhanced sonography for differential diagnosis of pleurisy and focal pleural lesions of unknown cause. Chest. 2005;128:3894–9.
14. Gorg C, Bert T, Kring R. Contrast enhanced sonography of peripheral lung lesions. AmJ Roentgenol. 2006;187:420–9.
15. Gorg C, Bert T, Kring R, et al. Transcutaneous contrast enhanced sonography of the chest for evaluation of pleural based pulmonary lesions: experience in 137 patients. Ultraschall Med. 2006;27:437–44.
16. Bard R, editor. Image guided dermatologic treatment. Berlin: Springer; 2019.
17. Chakr R, Santos J, Avles L, et al. Ultrasound assessment of disease activity prevents disease-modifying antirheumatic drug (DMARD) escalation and may reduce DMARD-related direct costs in rheumatoid arthritis with fibromyalgia. J Ultrasound Med. 2020;39:1271–8.
18. Kripfgans O, Pinter S, Baiu C, et al. Three-dimensional US for quantification of volumetric blood flow: multisite multisystem results from within the quantitative imaging biomarkers alliance. Radiology. 2020;296(3):671–82. https://doi.org/10.1148/radiol.2020191332.

Multimodality 3D Lung Imaging

8

Robert L. Bard

8.1   Introduction

As a member of the European Society of Radiology, Sociedad Espanola de Ecografia and Editorial Advisor to the Journal of Ultrasound (Rome) I had a front row seat to the ongoing progression of the Covid-19 pandemic and was privileged to communicate electronically with the treating physicians since February 2020. Other than the usual advantages of lung imaging with ultrasound (US)—ease of use, portability, lack of ionizing radiation, ability to sanitize—is the facts that CT is not a screening tool for Covid-19 pneumonia and the lab tests still have false positives. Screening is important since 50% of patients entering the emergency room do not present with fever [1]. As medicine reviews the many surprises that we have seen in the first year of this pandemic, it is relevant to consider the time honored acceptance of the stethoscope for lung diagnosis. While the emergency and intensive care clinicians have adopted point of care (POC) lung ultrasound as the first line of diagnosis, older physicians and most other colleagues are reluctant to use this technology. Part of the reason is the cost of the POC unit (from 2000 to 50,000 USD) compared with the $100–$300 stethoscope already in the lab coat. Also the learning curve for lung ultrasound depends on the imaging background of the clinician; however, medical students with 18 h of cardiac ultrasound training (programs have been on ongoing since 2012) are more accurately diagnosing heart problems with POC units than experienced cardiologists with their stethoscopes.

R. L. Bard (✉)
Bard Diagnostics, New York, NY, USA
e-mail: rbard@cancerscan.com

8.2   Stethoscopic Accuracy (Table 8.1)

Aside from accuracy and specificity, stethoscopes are known to carry *Staphylococcus aureus* and MRSA bacteria and have already been linked to a Covid-19 outbreak in a South African hospital. According to the 7/15/2020 Statnews.com article, the majority of stethoscopes "are cleaned rarely or never." Many of this year's POC units can be carried in the pocket much like the conventional stethoscope and probably will replace them for presumable infectious acute care patients. These are listed in the Appendix.

8.3   Lung Sonogram Indications

Indications for an ultrasound examination of the lung (including diaphragm, pleura, and rib cage structures) include but are not limited to:

- Dyspnea;
- Respiratory failure;
- Undifferentiated shock;
- Suspicion of pneumothorax;
- Assessment of the volume status;
- Assessment for pleural effusions;
- Evaluation for the presence of alveolar consolidation;
- Diaphragmatic function;
- Assessment of chest wall intercostal muscle contraction;
- Abnormal blood gases or other laboratory findings consistent with lung pathology;
- Thoracic trauma (focused assessment with sonography for trauma);
- Pleural-based masses;
- Planning or guidance for an invasive thoracic procedure.

Table 8.1 Stethoscopic accuracy in various clinical conditions

Condition	Auscultation		POC ultrasound	
	Sensitivity	Specificity	Sensitivity	Specificity
Pulmonary edema-congestive heart failure	46%	67%	97%	98%
Asthma/COPD	30%	90%	89%	97%
Pleural effusion—200 cc or more	42%	90%	100%	100%
Pleural effusion—less than 200 cc	Not detect	Not detect	93%	96%

8.3.1 Normal Lung Exam

The normal findings in supine, recumbent, prone, or erect position demonstrate a lung sliding motion on B-mode with a characteristic appearance on both A-mode and M-mode. Structures encountered from the skin surface are: dermis (epidermis with higher resolution probes), subcutaneous tissues, pectoral muscles, rib (anterior rib shows centrally echogenic costal cartilage), intercostal muscles (with lateral thoracic and/or internal mammary arteries on Doppler), and pleural line (Figs. 8.1, 8.2, and 8.3). Dynamic examination may be performed for accuracy of questionable structures since the intercostal muscles will contract and expand during respiration, which may be measured by M-mode. This may be later compared with post-ventilation atrophy and used as a visual guide for patients to accelerate respiratory therapies (Fig. 8.4).

8.3.2 A-Line Artifacts

A lines are seen in normally aerated lungs as reverberation artifacts appearing as linear horizontal echogenic smooth lines reflecting off the intact visceral pleural lining–normal lung interface. These bright white bands are displayed and repeated uniformly in evenly spaced intervals from the pleural line to the bottom of the image. A reduced gain setting makes the distinctive line pattern clearer in a noisy scan field. These repetitive lines are specific since the distance from the skin to the pleura line equals the distance from the pleural line to the first A-line and from the initial A-line to the second and successive interval A-lines. A-lines disappear as lung pathology increases and reappear as the pulmonary parenchyma–pleural interface normalizes. These physiologic appearances vary with transducer selection, probe placement, angulation and respiratory dynamics (Figs. 8.5, 8.6, and 8.7).

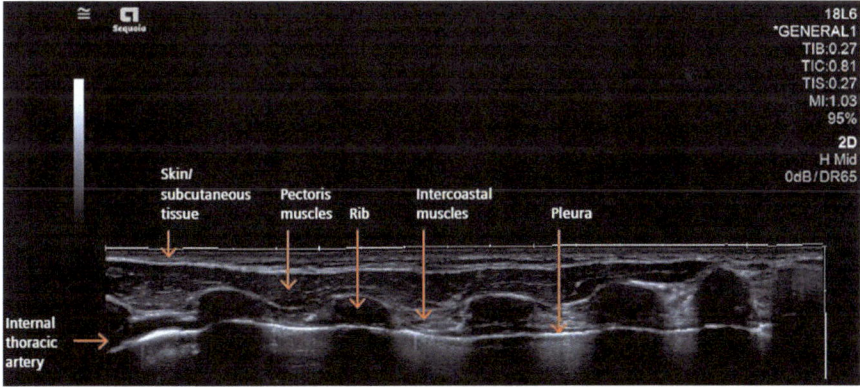

Fig. 8.1 Anatomical basics of the superficial chest wall structures and lung using the panoramic view

Fig. 8.2 Anatomical basics of the chest wall structures and the internal thoracic artery using the color Doppler examination

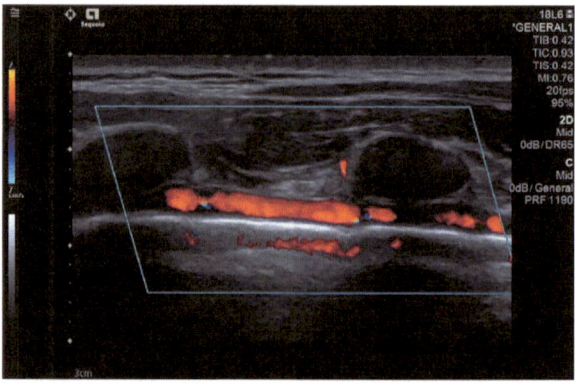

Fig. 8.3 Dynamic examination of the intercostal muscles. Relaxation of the muscle during expiration

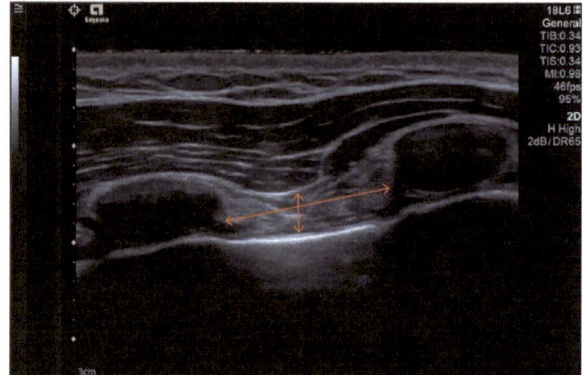

8.3.3 B-Line Artifacts

Sonographic patterns of these artifactual reverberations are termed B-lines and are hyperechoic linear echoes arising from the pleural line extending vertically to the bottom of the image. These dynamic artifactual lines are generated by increased or accumulated interstitial fluid and often appear at the lung bases or diaphragmatic–pleural interface in elderly or bed ridden patients as an incidental finding if no more than two in a particular field of view. Comet tail artifacts are fading short echoes not to be mistaken for a true "B-line" (Fig. 8.8). The radiologic CT correlation of B-lines generated by interstitial disease is the "lung rocket" and the radiographic image of alveolar fluid correlates with the ground glass opacity finding best seen on high resolution CT (GGO). B-lines may be present as single, multiple or confluent filling the entire screen. Often the pleural line will be less echogenic and thickened or irregular. To best appreciate B-lines one follows the A-lines until they disappear or map the B-lines until the A-lines reappear. This is advisable to more clearly evaluate abnormal pleural findings as the transition comparison is distinct (Figs. 8.9 and 8.10).

Fig. 8.4 Dynamic
examination of the
intercostal muscles.
Contraction of the muscle
during inspiration

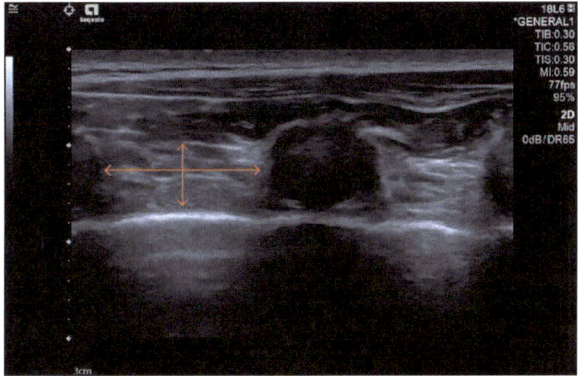

Fig. 8.5 Ultrasound image
demonstrating A-lines
using a linear transducer.
The A-lines are the bright
horizontal lines deep to the
pleural line. A-lines are a
classic reverberation
artifact

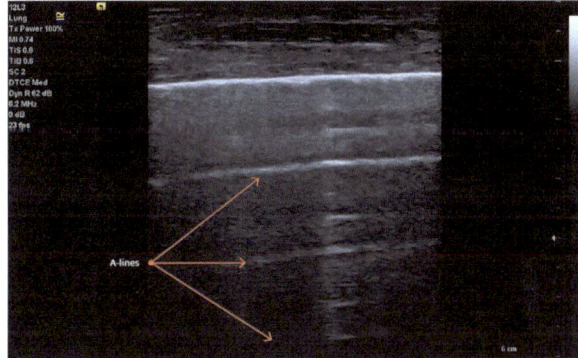

8.3.4 C-Line Artifacts

This pattern is a reverberation artifact generated by visceral pleura sliding over parietal pleura creating intermittent millimeter echogenic foci. When the pleural surfaces are in contact the rubbing artifact looks like ants crawling on the screen. The
presence of C-lines rules out pneumothorax and is important when respiratory
motion is severely restricted or absent. The sliding motion appears to "crawl" across
the field of view in real time and resembles ants moving in a line.

8.3.5 Lung Sliding

Lung sliding is visible during physiologic respiration as a to and fro or back and
forth movement. The margin of the pneumothorax (point of visceral pleural separation from the parietal pleura) with the normal lung is called the lung point at which
location the sliding motion ceases. Presence of a lung point indicates that air or
pneumothorax is absent in the scanned region. On M-mode a characteristic echo
pattern that looks like a bar code and has been called the "stratosphere sign."
Emergency image interpretation based on the presence of lung sliding starts with

Fig. 8.6 Ultrasound image demonstrating A-lines using a curved transducer. The A-lines are the bright horizontal lines deep to the pleural line. A-lines are a classic reverberation artifact. The distance from the skin to the pleural line equals the distance from the pleural line to the first A-line

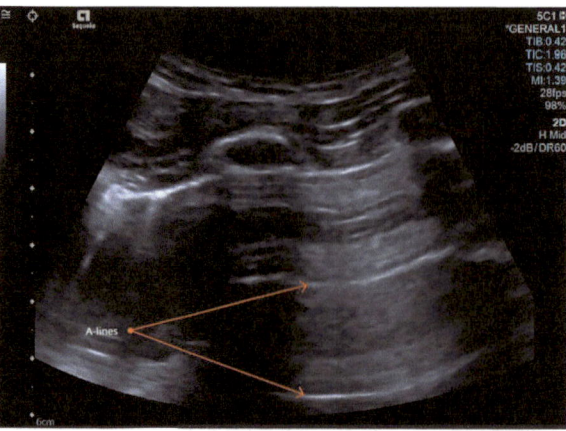

Fig. 8.7 Ultrasound image demonstrating A-lines using a curved transducer. The A-lines are clearly visible on the M-mode as bright white lines

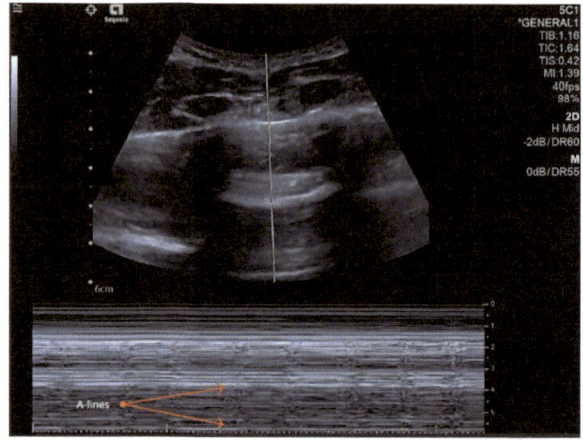

the presence or absence of this sign. If present, uniformly we look at the B-line profile for pulmonary edema or the A-line profile to see if deep vein imaging is called on to find thrombosis leading to pulmonary embolism. Normal venous imaging suggests presence of pneumonia or COPD or asthma. Abolished lung sliding indicates observation of the B-line profile for pneumonia or the A-line profile to check for a lung point indicating pneumothorax. Absent sliding without lung point needs further diagnostic modalities. Pneumonia may show A-lines, B-lines, C-lines in any pattern depending on the area insonated by a particular probe.

8.3.6 Lung Pulse

Lung pulse is the rhythmic pulsation of the pleura with adjacent cardiac contraction, which may be observed with greatly diminished respiratory excursion. The presence of intermittent C-lines indicates absence of pneumothorax. The finding of lung

Fig. 8.8 Ultrasound image demonstrating comet tail artifacts. The artifact originates at the pleura but fades

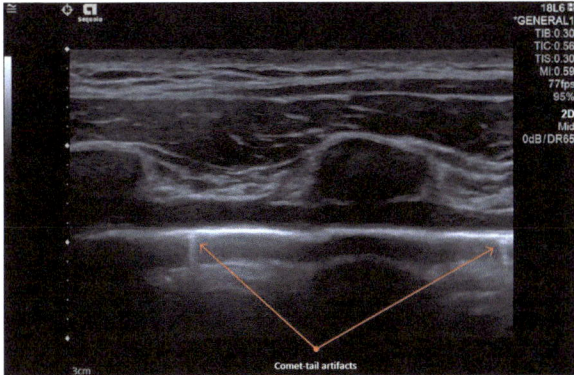

Fig. 8.9 Examination of the lung using a linear transducer. B-lines are discrete vertical hyperechoic reverberation artifacts that arise from the pleural line and extend to the bottom of the screen without fading. These artifacts move synchronously with lung sliding

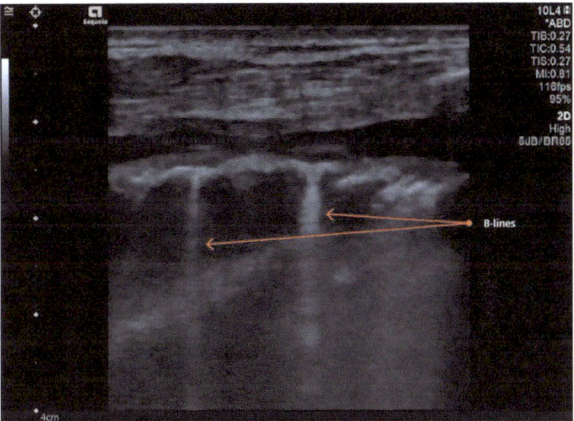

sliding is 100% sensitive for the exclusion of pneumothorax present at a given inter-space. Multiple rib interfaces should be examined if the suspicion of pneumothorax is high. A small apical pneumothorax may be missed because of shadowing from bone. If the presence of lung sliding is unclear in a patient with a high pretest prob-ability, a further evaluation should be performed [1, 2]. When this pattern is present, pneumothorax cannot be ruled out. Examples of disease processes that cause loss of lung sliding without pneumothorax include pleurodesis, severe emphysema with bullous lung disease, a severe acute respiratory distress syndrome pattern, opposing main-stem intubation, and apnea [3–8].

8.4   Pleural Ultrasound

Indications for pleural ultrasound include but are not limited to:

- Dyspnea;
- Evaluation for the presence, size, and complexity of pleural effusions;

Fig. 8.10 Examination of the lung using a curved transducer. B-lines are seen arising from the pleural line and extending to the bottom of the screen without fading

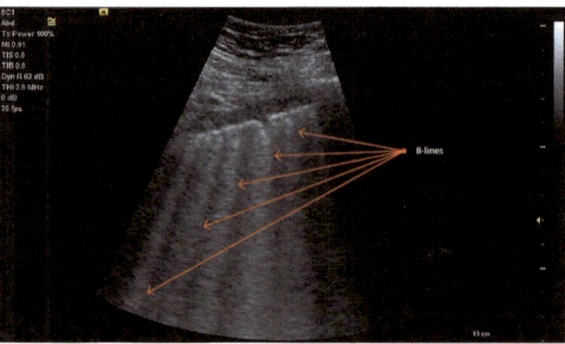

- Evaluation for the presence of hemothorax;
- Evaluation of the thickness and irregularity of the pleural line;
- Suspicion of interstitial lung disease;
- Evaluation of pneumothorax; and.
- Determination of the lung point.

Pleural disorders in the near field are best scanned with the linear probe while deeper effusions are better imaged with the curved or phased array probes. The probe angle should be adjusted to a true perpendicular plane to the pleural interface. The pleural line or visceral pleura–lung interface is the starting location for lung diagnosis and the presence of artifacts from other acute or chronic pulmonary disorders may appear as "comet tail artifacts" which arise from pleural pathologies. These may be difficult to distinguish from B-lines but are usually associated with parietal or visceral pleural thickening best appreciated with the linear probe or the higher resolution 3D/4D volumetric transducers. In the Covid-19 lung the pleural line may be irregular and fragmented or interrupted and thickened. In patients with COPD or collagen/interstitial diseases the comet tail sign is generally associated with a smooth pleural line. Pleural and subpleural hypoechoic regions or small foci of echo free pleural effusion indicated that the disease is worsening. In general, inflammatory pleura is thicker and more irregular than noninflamed pleural surfaces. The B-line pattern can be present in, but not specific to, cardiogenic and noncardiogenic pulmonary edema. The thickness of the pleura and the location of the B-line pattern may aid in the differentiation of these two disease processes (Fig. 8.11). The clinician may be able to differentiate between atelectasis and pneumonia causing the consolidation process. This is a clinical distinction, but the presence of mobile/dynamic air bronchograms indicates a bronchus that is patent [9].

8.4.1 Probe Positions

Protocol for basic scanning is four quadrants right and left lung:
  Quadrant 1 mid-clavicle upper lung Quadrant 2 mid-clavicle lower lung.
  Quadrant 3 mid-axilla upper lung Quadrant 4 mid-axilla lower lung (Fig. 8.12).

Fig. 8.11 Pneumonia examination of the lung with a linear transducer. Ultrasound findings including pleural effusion, pleural thickening and consolidations with additional accompanying B-line artifacts are seen

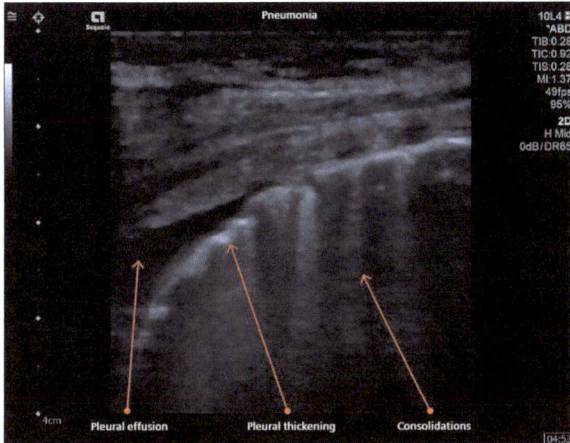

Fig. 8.12 Transducer positions for a lung ultrasound examination in the recumbent/supine patient. The abbreviated examination covers two BLUE points and the PLAPS (posterolateral alveolar and/or pleural syndrome) points on both sides (for the detailed description and how to localize BLUE and PLAPS points

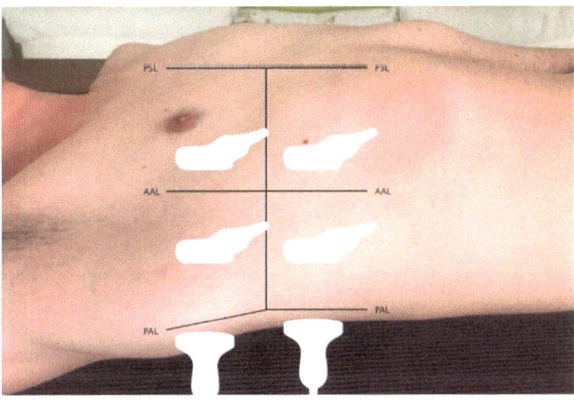

Additional views are obtained by erect posterior images and subcostal scans that show the inferior and posterior segments and provide motion analysis of the diaphragm and appear in other chapters as recommended by other authors.

8.5 Consolidation

8.5.1 Pneumonia

This is finding is visualized in cases of pneumonia, lung cancer, atelectasis, pulmonary infarction, lung contusion and ARDS. Since these are most often found in the posterior peripheral segments of the lung fields, a curved array probe images the pleural lining and still penetrate to find deeper effusions and consolidations. Tissue harmonic imaging (THI) is useful in penetrating the liver like gray-colored consolidated lung parenchyma called "hepatization" of the pulmonary tissue. Linear array

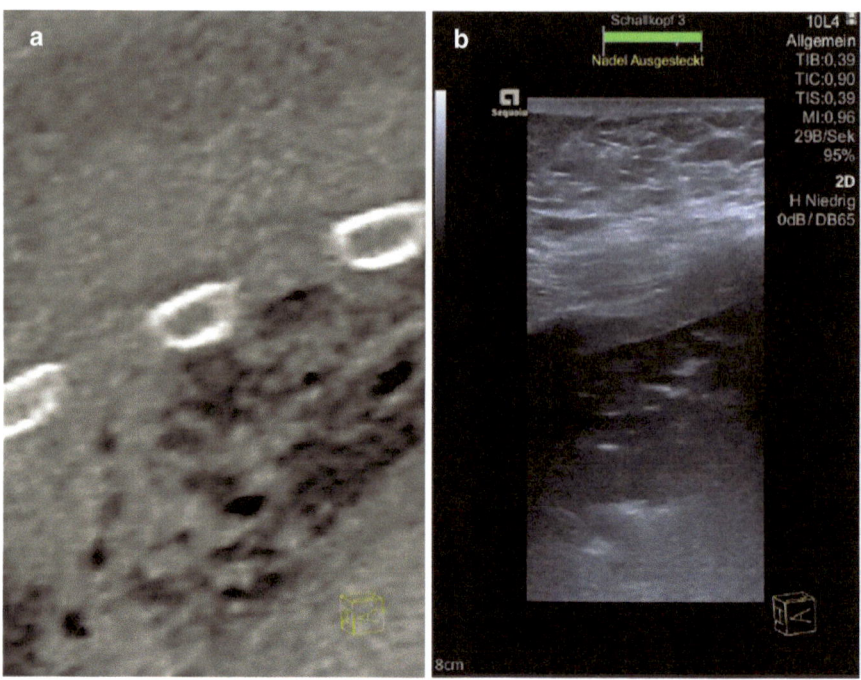

Fig. 8.13 Covid-19 pneumonia. Follow-up examination in the ICU using real-time image fusion technique with a linear transducer. HR-CT showed large flaps of soft tissues and low-density shadows under the pleura in the posterior segment of upper lobe of the left lung, and a large air bronchogram sign confirmed by ultrasound using the image fusion technique

probes require posterior probe positioning for most lower lobe disease which may be difficult to image in the acutely ill patient (Figs. 8.13a, b and 8.14a–d).

Findings demonstrate irregular nonhomogeneous echogenic tissue like echo pattern to the lung that simulates the liver echo structures and is termed "lung hepatization." B-lines in the area are nonhomogeneous and air bronchograms may be present due to residual air in the bronchi and have a "starry sky" appearance due to the echogenic air–bronchus interface. There are two types of air bronchograms: static and dynamic; static air bronchograms due to trapped residual air move with respiration and are found in any type of lung consolidative disorder while dynamic air bronchograms from active residual air flow into and out of the bronchi look like moving speckles with inspiration and expiration suggestive of aeration suggestive more of inflammation as opposed to noninflammatory causes.

The increased through transmission of homogeneously consolidated translobar lung tissue gives rise to the "spine sign" where the sound wave penetrating and reflecting back from anterior vertebra due to the lack impeding lung aeration provides a ladderlike echo pattern also seen in large pleural effusions. When the inflamed fluid filled parenchyma is inhomogeneous and nontranslobar, the appearance of this fractile border artifact is called the "shred sign" due to ring down

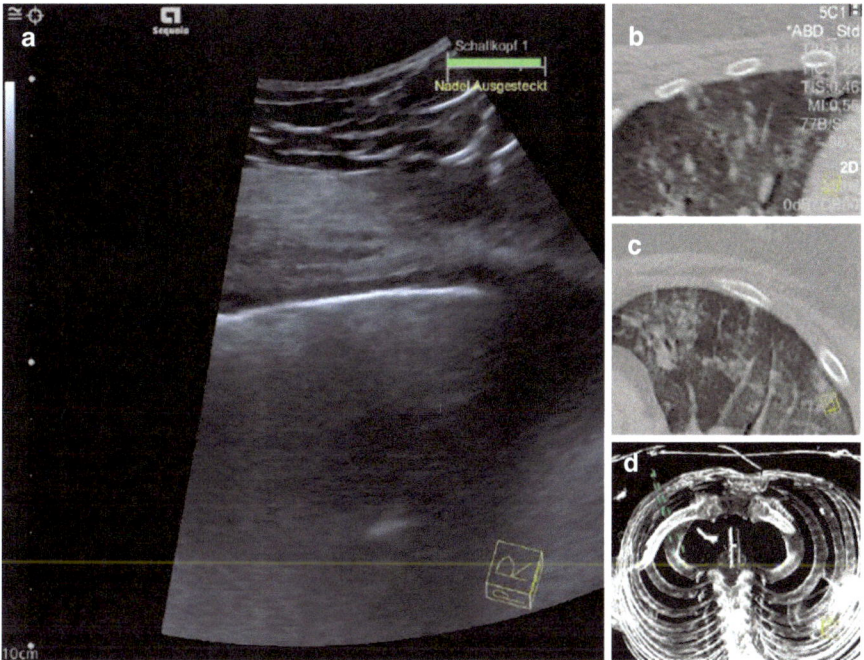

Fig. 8.14 Covid-19 pneumonia. Follow-up examination in the ICU using real-time image fusion technique with a curved transducer. Ultrasound findings including pleural thickening and consolidations of the lung in the side-by-side mode are detected. HR-CT showed ground glass opacity and reticular shadows under the pleura in the field of the right lung

reverberations that are intermittent and vary with respiratory phase. Accompanying atelectactic volume loss is noted by decreased size during inspiration due to recruitment. In the lower lungfields verification of the liver-diaphragmatic interface and splenic diaphragmatic interfaces are critical landmarks to distinguish liver and spleen from pulmonary consolidation especially in the presence of irregular fluid collections or empyema. Doppler flow dynamics of consolidated lung is present and not noted in pleural effusions unless complicated by loculated areas of neovascularity from acutely inflamed tissue or walls of malignant sheets due to aggressive tumor infiltration. The brightly echogenic findings from the tubular aerated bronchi are difficult to image on 2D planes so 3D reconstruction or 4D real time with Doppler better detects the branching pattern of bronchi or pulmonary vessels with these advanced technologies. The so called "lung pulse" from cardiac activity may be noted. When the patient is recovering, the use of these sophisticated imaging technologies may be used in the radiology suite as targeted 3D/4D volumetric image reproduction is generally obtained in seconds as opposed to many minutes with 2D scan protocols.

8.5.2   Doppler Flow Patterns

Doppler flow may differentiate the etiology in indeterminate cases. Pneumonia and atelectasis will have vessels with regular branching distribution while cancers demonstrate vessel irregularity and A-V fistulae. Chest wall vessels such as lateral thoracic artery and the internal mammary artery are echo free areas that must be identified before thoracentesis is considered. Pulsatility of the echofree area may be hard to visualize or related to lung pulse findings. Doppler and color flow Doppler US have shown decreased blood flow in these areas possibly due to edematous expanding tissue volume impeding the venous or arterial flow patterns in certain area which may be better understood when comparing the larger branching vascular pattern in a volumetric 3D/4D sonogram. Hematoma from contusion and pulmonary infarction shows absence of blood flow except in the periphery when neovascularization occurs. A B-line pattern can be present in, but not specific to, cardiogenic and noncardiogenic pulmonary edema. The thickness of the pleura and the location of the B-line pattern may aid in the differentiation of these two disease processes.

8.6   Pneumothorax

The air situated between the pleural surfaces creates the absence of lung sliding, A-lines, B-lines, C-lines, and lung pulse. The presence of a lung point further indicates a focal air collection with a predictive value approaching 100%. The finding of lung sliding or C-lines is 100% sensitive for the exclusion of pneumothorax present at a given interspace. Multiple rib interfaces should be examined if the suspicion of pneumothorax is high. A small apical pneumothorax may be missed because of shadowing from bone. Patient position flat-prone or supine-is preferred. If the presence of lung sliding is unclear in a patient with a high pretest probability, a further evaluation should be performed. Scans may be used concomitantly to monitor the position of a (CVC) central venous catheter without the use of a confirmatory X-ray (Fig. 8.15). M-mode is useful demonstrating an echogenic appearance simulating a

Fig. 8.15 CT-Topogram of a lung detected a pneumothorax on the right side which was afterward treated with a Bülau-Drainage

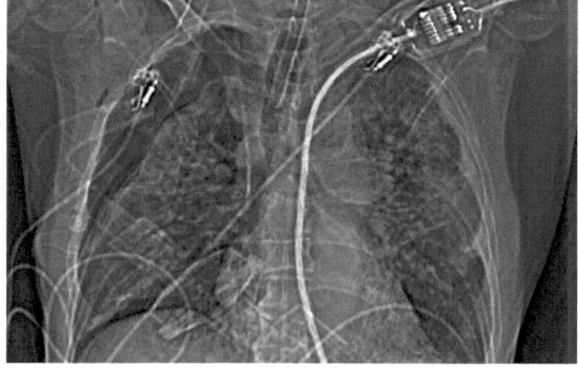

bar code or stratosphere appearance in diagnostically difficult areas since this may find air gap foci as small as 5 mm. Examples of disease processes that cause loss of lung sliding without pneumothorax include pleurodesis, severe emphysema with bullous lung disease, a severe acute respiratory distress syndrome pattern, opposing main-stem intubation, and apnea [3]. Rarely pneumothorax is complicated by the presence of pneumomediastinum (Figs. 8.16a, b, 8.17, 8.18, and 8.19).

8.7   Interstitial Syndrome

This entity is caused by pulmonary edema, interstitial pneumonia or pneumonitis, pulmonary fibrosis, ARDS, and diffuse parenchyma lung disease. Interstitial syndrome is a condition where alveolar aeration is impaired due to an increase in fluids in the pulmonary interstitium with some lung aeration preserved. B-lines are found in "interstitial syndrome" where excess fluid in the alveoli is adjacent to the pleural surface and creates linear artifactual vertical lines also called "comet tails or rockets" originating from the pleural line and extending to the bottom of the scan field which tend to move with the lung sliding. Multiple lines (greater than 2 per field are considered pathologic) correlate with the presence of extravascular lung water and disappear when fluid is removed by diuretics or dialysis and obliterate the normal A-line pattern.

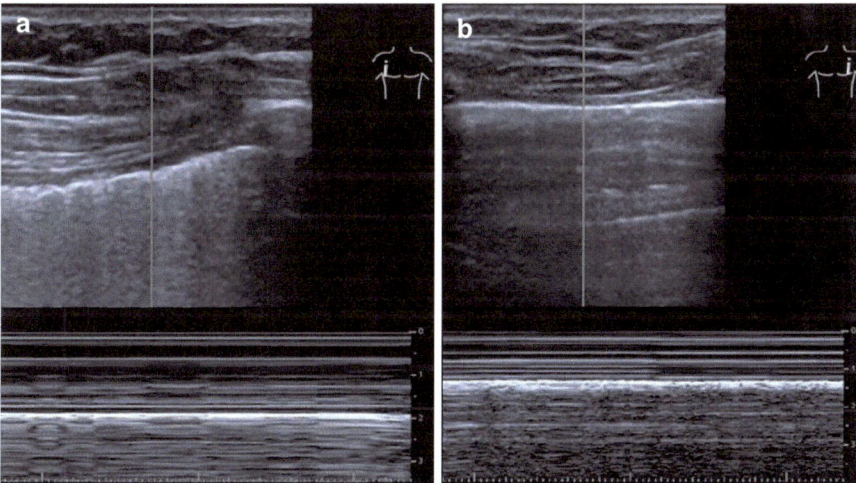

Fig. 8.16 Follow-up examination of the same patient two days later in the ICU. In M-mode (**a**), the absence of motion is documented as a static pattern of horizontal lines ("stratosphere sign"). In comparison to the M-mode (**b**), the seashore sign is clearly visible

Fig. 8.17 Covid-19 pneumonia. Follow-up examination in the ICU using a curved transducer. Ultrasound findings including pleural thickening and irregularity. Additionally, consolidations of the lung with B-lines are detected

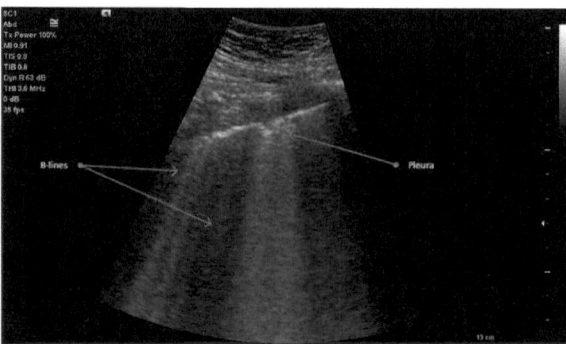

Fig. 8.18 Covid-19 pneumonia. Follow-up examination in the ICU using a sector transducer. Ultrasound findings including pleural thickening and irregularity. Additionally, consolidations of the lung with B-lines are detected

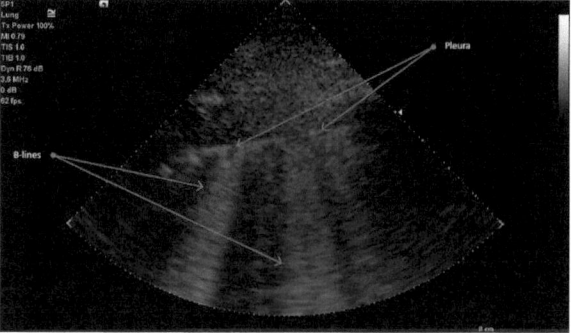

8.7.1 B-Line Pattern Recognition

In pulmonary edema, the B-lines tend to be diffusely homogeneous, usually bilateral, take up most of the lung surface and do not have skip areas when imaged. The distribution of B-lines also correlates with CT signs of fibrosis and lung sliding may be decreased due to the restrictive pulmonary process. B-lines in parenchymal lung disease are associated with pleural line abnormalities and subpleural abnormalities. ARDS images include anterior subpleural consolidations, reduction of lung sliding, "spared" areas of normal pulmonary parenchyma, nonhomogeneous B-line distribution and pleural line abnormalities. In severe cases, the confluence of B-lines may produce a white out effect that must be differentiate from lung consolidation. Diffuse interstitial pneumonia shows nonhomogenoeous B-line distribution, areas of spared lung and subpleural consolidations, foci of frank pulmonary consolidation and pleural line abnormalities.

8.8 Atelectasis

Collapsed lung is seen in many conditions but is uncommon in Covid without pleural effusion. This is more common in patients who are postoperative, bedridden or debilitated from diabetic or oncologic disorders. Lung sliding may be absent

Fig. 8.19 Covid-19 pneumonia. Follow-up examination in the ICU using a curved transducer. Ultrasound findings showed large areas of consolidation in the left posterior upper area and an air bronchogram sign

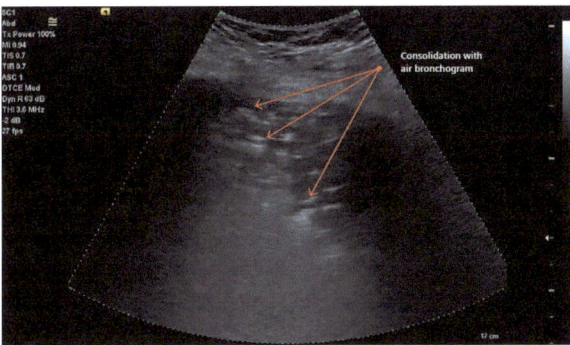

Fig. 8.20 Pleural effusion and slight dystelectasis of the left lower lobe

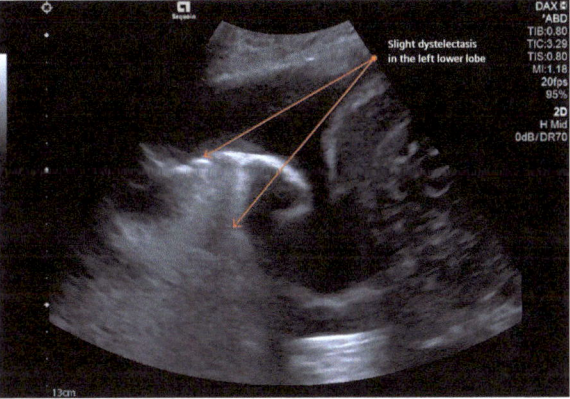

because the alveoli are not ventilated due to decreased or compressed lung volume and upward diaphragmatic dome displacement. The echogenicity is like liver ("lung hepatization") or splenic parenchyma in the case of complete atelectasis except for hyperechoic foci from partially aerated bronchioles. In infants, dystelectasis from partial collapse is more common. The clinician may be able to differentiate between atelectasis and pneumonia causing the consolidation process. This is a clinical distinction, but the presence of mobile/dynamic air bronchograms indicates a bronchus that is patent [9] (Fig. 8.20).

8.9   Pleural Effusion

Pleural effusions may be examined for size, complexity, and accessibility. The complexity of the fluid in hemothorax depends on the age of the collection. Complex effusions have stranding and debris indicative of inflammatory, infectious or malignant process. Diagnosis of a pleural effusion requires identification of anechoic or echogenic fluid with typical anatomic boundaries (chest wall, lung surface, and diaphragm) with associated dynamic findings (e.g., lung flapping, plankton sign, and diaphragmatic movement). In the supine patient, using a coronal view in the posterior axillary line, the spine sign should be sought to ensure that the anechoic region above the diaphragm is not erroneously present due to refraction artifacts. The pleural line should be examined for thickness, irregularity, and lung sliding in multiple rib interspaces [10]. Quantification or estimation of pleural effusion may be performed by using the methods of Balik et al. [11–14] or Remerand et al. using the formula $V = ME + DLX70$ ME = maximum effusion height, DL = distance from diaphragm base to the lung line of the visceral pleura. The "spine sign" is frequently present if the probe penetration depth is posterior, the fluid collection is posteriorly located and volume is sufficient to allow for higher through transmission of the sound waves. The "quad sign" is observed when the sagittal positioned probe images the appearance of a quadrangular space defined by the pleural line of the chest wall, the shadows of the ribs and the lung line of the visceral pleura (Figs. 8.21, 8.22, 8.23, 8.24, 8.25, 8.26, and 8.27).

8.10   Rib Cage

When scanning for pulmonary pathology, the ribs may be scanned for fracture (displaced or nondisplaced), chest wall adenopathy (malignant or inflammatory) and the presence of boney metastases which often accompanies malignant effusions that may be found in the elderly or patients with co-morbidities. Muscle abnormalities such as hematoma, fascial tear, and reduced contraction are observable. This is particularly true in anterior imaging where the echo free or echo poor costal cartilage may mimic a fluid collection or consolidation. M-mode and real-time video is useful in dynamically tracking the contraction and relaxation of the intercostal muscles during chest expansion with or without diaphragmatic assistance. Elastography may elicit the extent of fibrosis or fatty atrophy from prolonged ventilatory assistance. The pleural line is the starting location for lung diagnosis and the presence of artifacts from other acute or chronic pulmonary disorders may appear as comet tail artifacts, which arise from pleural pathologies. These may be difficult to distinguish from B-lines but are usually associated with parietal or visceral pleural thickening best appreciated with the linear probe or the higher resolution 3D/4D volumetric transducers.

Fig. 8.21 Pleural effusion right side

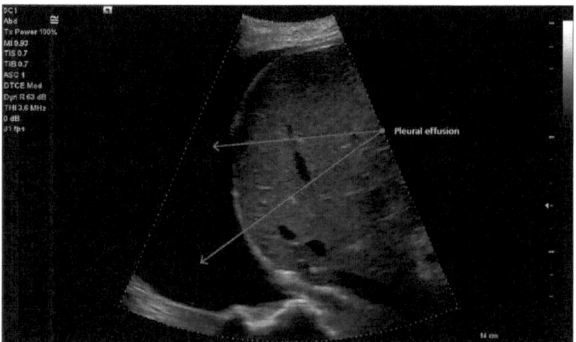

Fig. 8.22 Pleural effusion left side and adherent nodular structure to the diaphragm is detected

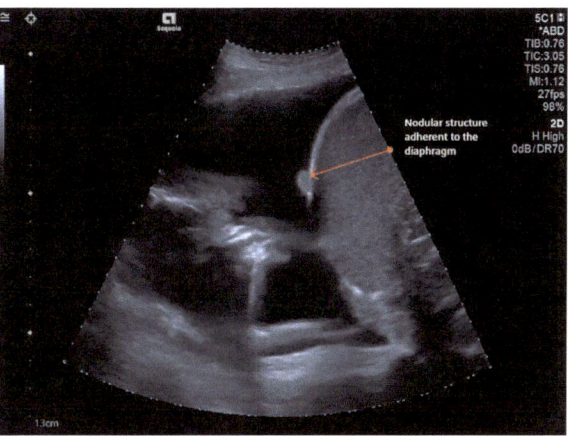

Fig. 8.23 Covid-19 pneumonia. Follow-up examination in the ICU using a curved transducer (5–1 MHz). Ultrasound findings including pleural thickening and irregularity. Additionally, consolidations of the lung with B-lines are detected

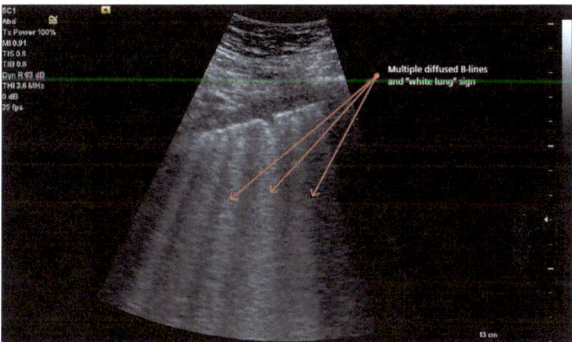

8.10.1 Probe Selection

Lung US ultrasound may be performed with a variety of probes since the mechanism of diagnosis is related to artifact generation and lesion location. The phased array "cardiac" transducer has low frequency and deep penetration. Doppler capability is an adjunct to performing cardiac flow analysis, IVC status observation and investigating blood flow in areas of consolidation. The curvilinear "abdominal" transducer is low frequency with greater depth penetration. This general purpose probe affords rapid evaluation of many areas with good accuracy. The linear "vascular" transducer is high frequency with greater resolution and shallower penetration. Wireless probes are useful and single focal point with focus on the pleural line is optimal for pleural imaging. A low mechanical index (MI) for starting and lowering if possible while optimizing a low gain setting. High frame rate while avoiding settings such as harmonics, Doppler and contrast (unless indicated) and compounding is suggested. Video storage clips are 2–4 s in each zone should accompany B-scan documentation.

The differences in acoustic impedance between air and water layers generate characteristic artifactual echo patterns. Normal lung is almost entirely air and the

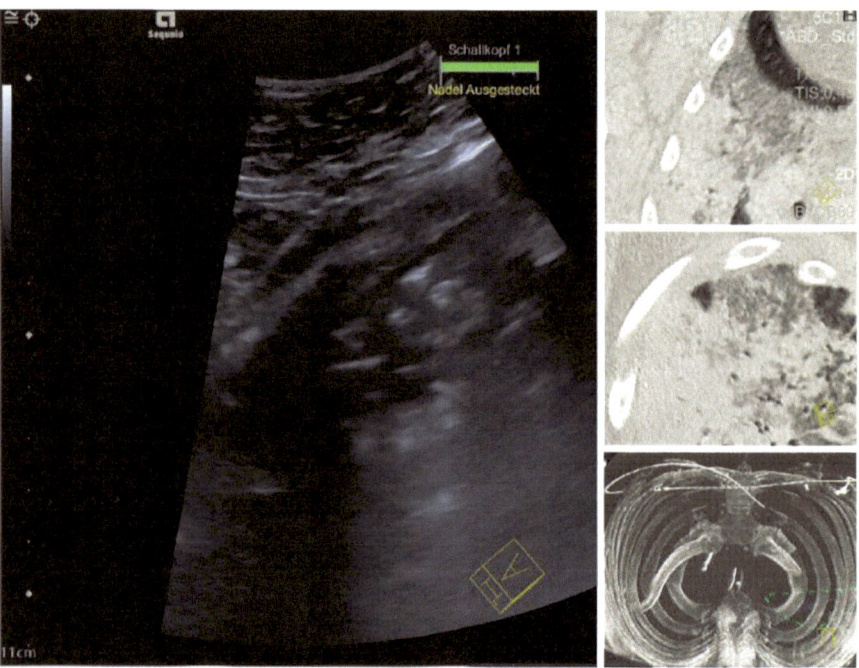

Fig. 8.24 Covid-19 pneumonia. Follow-up examination in the ICU using a curved transducer (5–1 MHz) and the image fusion technique. Ultrasound findings showed large areas of consolidation and an air bronchogram sign

Fig. 8.25 Covid-19 pneumonia. Follow-up examination in the ICU using a linear (12–3 MHz) transducer. Ultrasound findings including pleural thickening and irregularity are seen

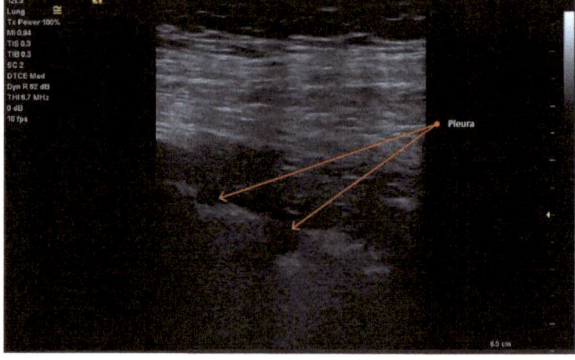

artifacts are generated at the pleural–lung interface. A-lines are repetitive horizontal echoes appearing as hyperechoic (bright) lines starting about 5 mm below the rib line and diminish in brightness as the depth increases which retaining the even interspacing. The normal pleural line is thin, homogeneous, and flat with sliding noticeable during respiration appearing as dots or interruptions in the smooth surface. Below the normal pleura is the typical artifact on M-mode that shows the lung sliding as inhomogeneous mid-level echoes often termed the "sandy beach sign."

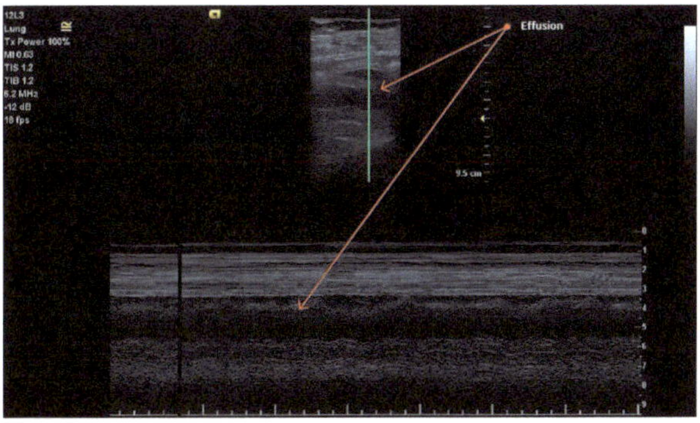

Fig. 8.26 Covid-19 pneumonia. Follow-up examination in the ICU using a linear (12–3 MHz) transducer including M-mode and B-mode ultrasound findings detected pleural thickening and an additional small pleural effusion

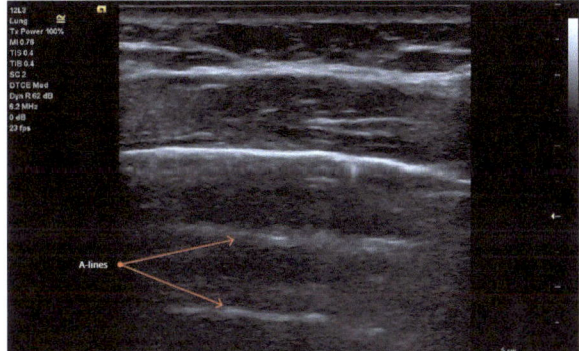

Fig. 8.27 Follow-up after artificial respiration of Covid-19 pneumonia on a patient in the ICU. An indirect sign for recovering is the appearance of A-lines during the recovery phase

8.10.2 Triage Imaging

Probe(s) selection may be based on the analysis of lung sliding normally visible during physiologic respiration as a to and fro movement. The margin of the pneumothorax (point of visceral pleural separation from the parietal pleura) with the normal lung is called the lung point at which location the sliding motion ceases. Presence of a lung point indicates that air or pneumothorax is absent in the scanned region. On M-mode a characteristic echo pattern that looks like a bar code and has been called the "stratosphere sign." Emergency image interpretation based on the presence of lung sliding starts with the presence or absence of this sign. If present uniformly we look at the B-line profile for pulmonary edema or the A-line profile to see if deep vein imaging is called on to find thrombosis leading to pulmonary embolism. Normal venous imaging suggests presence of pneumonia or COPD or asthma. Abolished lung sliding indicates observation of the B-line profile for pneumonia or the A-line profile to check for a lung point indicating pneumothorax. Absent sliding without lung point needs further diagnostic modalities. Pneumonia may show A-lines, B-lines, C-lines in any pattern depending on the area insonated by a particular probe. Lung pulse is the rhythmic pulsation of the pleura with adjacent cardiac contraction, which may be observed with greatly diminished respiratory excursion. The presence of intermittent C-lines indicates absence of pneumothorax.

8.11   Pitfalls in Scanning

Lung ultrasound relies on the images produced by artifacts. Many of the radiologic units and some of the newer point of care portable devices use advanced features to reduce artifactual generation such as compound imaging, speckle reduction and harmonics. These applications mask artifact generation and imaging is often improved by turning off these presets. Reduction of gain and dynamic range is useful for all probes. Curved, linear and phased array probes are optimized by customizing personal scan parameters to adjust to the clinical setting. Scan depth for curved and phased array probes is usually 8–14 cm while linear probes are optimized between 6 and 10 cm for adults. Scan depth is optimized by the area under investigation with the focus adjusted for example 5–9 mm depth for the anterior chest. A clear pleural line and appropriate A-line or B-line artifacts ensures proper probe position. A nonperpendicular plane scan produces anechoic regions that may be mistaken for a deep pleural effusion or a pneumothorax. In emergency scanning, the presence of a "bat sign" is a starting point to ensure the white horizontal lines are truly the rib-pleural–lung interface. The sonic shadow of the ribs with pleural echoes sandwiched in between may be likened to bat-wings with the echogenic chest wall as the body of the bat.

Absence of lung sliding may be due to COPD with or without emphysema, lung bullae, apnea, status post-pleurodeisis, high ventilator settings, mainstream intubation, and similar conditions such as severe asthma. Check for a subtle lung pulse to rule out pneumothorax and make sure the transducer is not placed over a rib. Tension pneumothorax with no pleural sliding will not disclose the important lung point artifact necessitating further imaging. A pseudo lung point occurs where the pericardium intermittently touches the visceral pleura. Misinterpreting situational findings such as expected conditions in a specific patient population, like small posterior effusions and dependent B-lines in the bedbound patient. In thin patients, the costal cartilage is often echo poor and may simulate subpleural consolidation. Higher frequency probes will show the true pleural line immediately adjacent to the rib margin and may differentiate the cartilaginous homogeneous echo pattern with increased through transmission.

8.12   Limitations of Lung Ultrasound

Ultrasound may be limited in the dyspneic, febrile, or trauma patient because of obesity, subcutaneous emphysema, patient positioning, the degree of injury, adhesions from prior surgery, and often patients who are either in pain, uncooperative or combative. The main limitation of the point-of-care thoracic examination is that the operator must be knowledgeable in its clinical use and aware of antiviral precautions.

Limitations of a point-of-care thoracic examination in the evaluation for pneumothorax include main-stem bronchus intubation, failure to recognize the lung pulse (subtle cardiac pulsation of the parietal pleura at the lung periphery) as cardiac-induced movement, patients after pleurodesis, and patients with severe chronic obstructive pulmonary disease or other lung pathology inhibiting adequate visualization of lung sliding. Although sensitivity in the detection of pneumothorax is very high, it is important to note that small apical pneumothorax or small localized pneumothoraces may not be visualized even in a carefully targeted thoracic ultrasound examination.

Limitations in the evaluation of the B-line pattern include the ability to differentiate between cardiogenic and noncardiogenic pulmonary edema producing a similar appearance. Limitations in the evaluation of a consolidation pattern include body habitus and failure to place the transducer in the posterior thorax to detect a posteriorly located consolidation. Limitations in the evaluation of Doppler flow in the consolidation include patient motion (body and diaphragmatic) and lack of B flow capability.

Ultrasound may be limited in the dyspneic, febrile or trauma patient because of obesity, subcutaneous emphysema, patient positioning, the degree of injury, adhesions from prior surgery, and often patients who are either in pain, uncooperative or combative. The main limitation of the point-of-care thoracic examination is that the operator must be knowledgeable in its clinical use and aware of antiviral precautions.

Limitations of a point-of-care thoracic examination in the evaluation for pneumothorax include main-stem bronchus intubation, failure to recognize the lung pulse (subtle cardiac pulsation of the parietal pleura at the lung periphery) as cardiac-induced movement, patients after pleurodesis, and patients with severe chronic obstructive pulmonary disease or other lung pathology inhibiting adequate visualization of lung sliding. Although sensitivity in the detection of pneumothorax is very high, it is important to note that small apical pneumothorax or localized pneumothoraces may not be visualized even in a carefully targeted thoracic ultrasound examination.

Limitations in the evaluation of the B-line pattern include the ability to differentiate between cardiogenic and noncardiogenic pulmonary edema producing a similar appearance. Limitations in the evaluation of a consolidation pattern include body habitus and failure to place the transducer in the posterior thorax to detect a posteriorly located consolidation. Limitations in the evaluation of Doppler flow in the consolidation include patient motion (body and diaphragmatic) and lack of B flow capability.

The many cosmetic procedure on the breast and surrounding areas may cause artifacts by: Unrecognized subdermal cysts or subdermal calcific foci especially in people following cosmetic procedures such and fillers and reconstructive surgeries. Postop seromas, misplaced cosmetic filler or relocated silicone deposits, air spaces from surgical trauma present obstacles to image interpretation. The rare complication of pneumomediastinum with or without pneumothorax in one or more sites would be a further limitation to correct image analysis. Air collections in resolving pulmonary hematoma or pneumomediastium (with or without pregnancy) cause unexpected scan images [15–17]. In cases of confusing findings, correlation with other imaging modalities is useful.

8.13   Limitations of Radiography

Since most cases will need to be correlated with X-ray or CT findings, it is important to note the limitations of X-ray and CT findings. X-ray misses most early Covid disease but is useful in finding the more advanced pneumonic consolidation process. Typical chest CT findings in Covid-19 pneumonia include bilateral, peripheral and basal-predominant ground glass opacities (GGOs) and/or consolidation, followed later by a mixed pattern of crazy paving, architectural distortion and perilobular abnormalities superimposed on GGOs that slowly resolve.

Upper lobe or peribronchovascular distribution of GGOs, cavitation, lymphadenopathy, and pleural thickening are found atypically and frank pneumonic consolidation is extremely rare in the pediatric population.

It is impossible to differentiate Covid-19 typical image findings from other diseases. For example, bacterial pneumonia can present with focal segmental or lobar pulmonary opacities without lower lung predominance, but other common findings (cavitation, lung abscess, lymphadenopathy, and so on) can usually differentiate it from Covid-19.

Other viral pneumonias are more challenging to distinguish from Covid-19. For example, ground glass opacities (GGOs) can be seen in up to 75% of adenovirus cases, more than 75% of cytomegalovirus and herpes simplex virus cases, and up to 25% of measles and human meta-pneumovirus cases.

GGOs can be widespread in pneumocystis pneumonia, but, unlike in Covid-19, they tend to predominate in the upper lobes. Similarly, various interstitial lung diseases can present with GGOs, but the predominant location differs by diagnosis, and other clinical factors are useful for differentiating them from Covid-19.

GGOs can also be common in hypersensitivity pneumonitis, lung injury from use of electronic cigarettes or vaping products, pulmonary edema, diffuse alveolar hemorrhage, pulmonary alveolar proteinosis, and eosinophilic pneumonia. But clinical features and GGO patterns are generally useful for differentiating these conditions from Covid-19.

CT is valuable in identifying underlying cardiopulmonary abnormalities in patients with moderate to severe disease. CT can help clinicians triage resources toward patients at risk of disease progression and may identify a cause in case of clinical worsening. CT may also identify alternate diagnoses.

Dr. Marcello Migliore of the University of Catania, in Italy, who recently reviewed the management of GGOs in the lung cancer screening era, told Reuters Health by email, "CT is not useful to diagnose Covid-19, but it is certainly useful to follow-up patients with preexisting lung pathology who go rapidly worse. However,

GGOs are also a presenting picture of early lung cancer and therefore it should be taken into account."

8.13.1 Best Practices

Adequate documentation is essential for high-quality patient care. Ultrasound images that contain diagnostic information and/or direct patient management (both normal and abnormal) should be recorded in accordance with the *AIUM Practice Parameter for Documentation of an Ultrasound Examination* [18].

8.13.2 Equipment Specifications

All studies should be performed at the point of care.

- For abdominal studies, phased array or curvilinear transducers are preferred; however, a higher-frequency linear transducer may be used. For adults, mean frequencies between 2 and 5 MHz are most commonly used. For most preadolescent pediatric patients, mean frequencies of 5 MHz or greater are preferred, and in neonates and small infants, a higher-frequency linear transducer is often necessary. For cardiac studies, phased array transducers are preferred. For pediatrics and adults, mean frequencies between 2 and 5 MHz are most commonly used. For DVT studies, equipment must be capable of real-time imaging for compression of the veins. In most cases, a linear or curvilinear transducer is preferable, but phased array scanners can be helpful for difficult patients. Transducers should transmit at a frequency of 5 MHz or greater, with the occasional need for a lower-frequency transducer. Color Doppler imaging and spectral Doppler flow analysis can be used to augment the examination.
- For thoracic studies, phased array, curvilinear, and higher-frequency linear transducers are preferable; all may be used, with the preference varying based on the clinical question to be answered. For adults, mean frequencies between 2 and 5 MHz are generally used.

The equipment should be adjusted to operate at the highest clinically appropriate frequency, realizing that there is a trade-off between resolution and beam penetration. When Doppler studies are performed, the Doppler frequency may differ from the imaging frequency. Image quality should be optimized while keeping total ultrasound exposure as low as reasonably achievable. Phased array, curvilinear, and higher-frequency linear transducers are preferable; all may be used, with the preference varying based on the clinical question to be answered. For adults, mean frequencies between 2 and 5 MHz are recommended.

The equipment should be adjusted to operate at the highest clinically appropriate frequency, realizing that there is a trade-off between resolution and beam penetration. When Doppler studies are performed, the Doppler frequency may differ from the imaging frequency. Image quality should be optimized while keeping total ultrasound exposure as low as reasonably achievable (ALARA).

8.14   Image Fusion

Cross-sectional interventional procedures are performed under CT, ultrasound, fluoroscopy, or MRI guidance and include fluid aspiration, (thoracentesis, paracentesis, and fluid collections), drainage catheter placement, percutaneous biopsy, and tumor ablation. Fusion applications make advanced treatments clinically viable. Image fusion for biopsy of the prostate combining ultrasound and MRI images has been widely adapted since 2012 in the United States. In Europe, chest fusion studies began in 2005 and become widely used about 10 years later. Fusion of MRI, PET-CT, PET-MRI or MS-CT chest images may be facilitated in the ICU by accessing previous radiology department data and merging this with the current ultrasound images to see if the consolidation existed in the past. The possible contraindication is a cardiac pacemaker for since the fusion process involving the placement of magnetic markers used as sensors for the transducer motion placement. DICOM data from the past CT exam (or possible previous MRI) is downloaded into the fusion system for comparison with the current US study. Linear or curved probes may be used to create the field of US scan that is generated from the CT image and then fused. These findings may be compared with 3D/4D US volumetric imaging as well. Recovering patients have decreased blood flow in areas of improving lung consolidation. Artificial intelligence and advanced algorithms are being developed to generate a real-time scoring system and segmentation of LUS data. However useful in the future, given the rapidly dynamic changes with this disease and multiorgan involvement, the best clinical use is to document either a normal lung scan or imaging findings that are improving or accelerating at given time intervals that may be based on changes in oxygen saturation levels [19, 20].

Fusion of medical imaging involves combining multiple images from either the same patient or multiple patients. These images may be MRI, CT, and ultrasound, or various parameters from different MRI or CT scans of a single patient. Since each different image may offer orthogonal information, fusing these images allows clinicians to make a more informed diagnosis (in the case of fusing CT/MRI parameters), or in using an MRI or CT to more precisely guide an ultrasound biopsy toward a tumor target or to use a sonogram to guide a CT image guided procedure. For example, fusion could allow clinicians to take advantage of previously captured images, merged with real-time ultrasound, to gain enhanced information about suspected tumors or focal inflammatory processes with a precision that transcends ultrasound or CT alone. However, fusion requires that these various images be brought into spatial alignment, a process referred to as computerized "registration." Several device manufacturers offer registration systems, but registration algorithms are still an area of active research. The sheer number of images being acquired daily by clinicians such as radiologists is staggering. These include Magnetic Resonance Imaging (MRI), Transrectal Ultrasound (TRUS), and Computerized Tomography

(CT) to name a few. Frequently, multiple imaging sequences are acquired from the same patient. In the case of MRI, multiple different parameters are acquired in the same scanning session, resulting in a plethora of images acquired within minutes of each other. Each type of imaging sequence may contain orthogonal information. For example, a T2-weighted MRI contains structural information, while Dynamic Contrast Enhanced (DCE) MRI contains the rate of contrast dye uptake by various vascularized regions within the body.

The amount of imaging information being acquired opens up an exciting possibility for doctors, as information from multiple sources can be used to make a more informed diagnostic or treatment decision. For example, a solid organ tumor may not be clearly visible on T2-weighted MRI, and yet can appear vivid on an Apparent Diffusion Coefficient (ADC) MRI image. However, a problem arises in that the various images are not necessarily spatially aligned. To make an informed decision as to whether a tumor is visible in a certain region of the prostate, the corresponding region must be realized on all the images. The process of bringing multiple images (from the same patient or different patients) into spatial alignment is the task known as "registration" and performed with the help of sophisticated computer vision algorithms.

8.14.1 Registration Overview

As stated previously, registration is the process of bringing multiple images into spatial alignment. The images are typically either 2D or 3D, although 4D time-series data is sometimes available. The goal of any registration algorithm is to determine a transformation which best aligns the images. This transformation can be as simple as translating the image (moving up/down, or left/right), or as sophisticated as warping certain spots within the images (called "deformable registration"). A computer algorithm essentially tries various transformations and finds the "optimal" one which best aligns the images. There is always a reference "fixed" image which does not move, and a "moving" image, to which the transformations are applied. Various transformations are tried, and an "interpolator" generates a "moved" image for each of those transformations. The "moved" image which most closely matches the "fixed" image is chosen (via the use of an "optimizer") and output. The following sections describe each of these processes in detail [21–24].

8.14.2 Transformations

A transformation is an integral component to any registration algorithm. It defines how to move, or deform, a given image. The two general categories of transformations are "linear" and "deformable" transformations. A linear transformation is any translation, rotation, scaling, or shearing which is applied to the image as a whole. A transformation which only allows translation and rotation is considered "rigid". When incorporating scaling and shearing, the transformation is considered "affine."

Rigid registration was used to fuse MRI and CT prostate images in Greene et al. A deformable registration allows warping of an image at specific locations. Essentially, in its most general form, every single pixel (or tiny location within the image with an intensity value) is allowed to move anywhere else in the image. There are various types of deformable transformations including B-Splines, Thin Plate Splines, and Finite Element Model transformations. Using a linear or deformable registration, a series of numbers is used to represent the given transformation. In the case of linear transformations, these numbers may represent the amount to translate the image (in mm), or the magnitude of rotation (in degrees). In the case of deformable registration, these numbers may represent how certain regions of the image should warp relative to other regions [25–29].

8.14.3 Interpolators

A given transformation is defined by a set of numbers, and an interpolator uses those numbers to generate a "moved" image. When stretching the image, for example, you don't want "holes" or "tears" to appear in the moved image. As such, the computer algorithm needs to decide how to stretch two adjacent regions of the image, and how to deal with regions, which lie between two pixels or result from stretching a pixel.

The following are the most common interpolators:

- **Nearest Neighbor**: The "nearest neighbor" interpolator is the simplest (and fastest) interpolator, in which the closest point on the moving image is chosen when deforming the image.
- **Linear**: The "linear" interpolator uses a linear blending of nearby pixel values to decide the color.
- **Spline**: A "spline" interpolator, similar to a linear interpolator, performs a blending of nearby pixel values. However, it fits a curve to the pixels and uses that to decide "how gray" to make the interpolated pixels. A spline interpolator may consider not just neighboring pixels, but also pixels a few mm away to make a more informed decision of the color. This interpolator typically takes much longer to compute than a linear interpolator, and may not necessarily yield a more accurate interpolation.

There are more sophisticated interpolators, but a tradeoff between computational time and accuracy leads most algorithms to employ a linear interpolator, as the marginal benefit of sophisticated interpolators rarely lead to a significant increase in registration accuracy [30–35].

8.14.4 Metrics

After interpolating a "moved" image, the algorithm then needs to compare this to the reference "fixed" image. This is done using a similarity metric, which yields a large number in the case of high similarity, and a low number in the case of a low similarity. This similarity is used to evaluate the correctness of a transform in registering the images. There are a plethora of similarity measures, which could be employed, and merits and issues with each. The most common ones in use for image registration are outlined below, although additional, more sophisticated measures have been developed for prostate registration [36–40].

- **Intensity Differences**: The differences in image intensity values are computed and summed over the entire image, or a region of the image [45]. For example, black may be given a value of 0, and white may be given a value of 1. If two pixels are spatially aligned and both have a value of white, then the difference could be 0. The algorithm typically will sum the absolute differences over all the pixels to output a final value, and negate that value (since we want to maximize, not minimize, the similarity). A value of 0 would indicate a perfectly spatially aligned image, and a large negative value would indicate an extremely dissimilar pair of images.
- **Normalized Cross Correlation (NCC)**: Using intensity differences is subject to various imaging artifacts such as changes in brightness and contrast, which could throw off the accuracy of the measure. In addition, one image may represent black with a value of 0, while another image may represent black with a value of 50, and as such the intensity differences may not be an accurate measure. The NCC between two images is a normalized measure calculated by fitting a line through a collection of pixel values in two images. Essentially if one image had intensity values of {20, 30, 40} at 3 pixels, and a second image had intensity values of {80, 90, 100} at those same 3 pixels, that would be considered perfectly aligned. This is mathematically similar to the intensity differences, but less prone to artifacts such as brightness and contrast.
- **Mutual Information (MI)**: MI is a more sophisticated measure derived from information theory. It essentially models how well the intensity values in one image can "predict" the intensity values in another image. MI quantifies the information content shared between two images, such that two images which share a lot of "information" get a high value (such as two prostate images from the same patient) and two images which share no information (such as a prostate and breast image) get a low value [41–44].

8.14.5 Optimizers

After computing the similarity of the moved and fixed images, and calculating the accuracy of the given transformation via the similarity metric, the algorithm must decide whether to try another transformation, or output the result.

The role of the optimizer is to (a) decide when the transformation is "good enough," and (b) decide what new transformation to try next. There are many different types of optimizers, and optimization is an area of active research. A few common optimizers employed in image registration are described below [45–47].

- **Simplex**: A simplex optimizer takes the previous transformation, and slightly modifies it based on the magnitude of the similarity error. It is one of the simplest optimizers, and may be useful in honing in on a transformation, but may not perform well in choosing an initial transformation.
- **Genetic Algorithm (GA)**: A GA optimizer for image registration considers each transformation as an "individual" in a population. It decides the relative "fitness" of each individual by the image similarity. Individuals (i.e., transformations) with low image similarity have a higher chance of dying out. Individuals with a high image similarity will mate and evolve over several generations. The underlying hypothesis is that only the fittest individuals (i.e., transformations with high image similarities) will remain after several generations.
- **Particle Swarm**: A particle swarm optimizer for image registration considers each transformation as a particle in space. A collection of particles represent various transformations and will have velocities proportional to their image similarities, and ideally converge on the optimal transformation.

Several common problems with optimizers is that (a) they may require a lot of parameters to tune, (b) may not necessarily know when to stop, and (c) can take a significant amount of computational time to arrive at a solution. This last issue is extremely important when one needs real-time registration, as in the case of MRI–TRUS fusion biopsy. Current research is attempting to address these issues in terms of both algorithmic improvements, and properly utilizing increases in computational power.

8.15   Acute Care Considerations

Imaging of the lung is divided into outpatient, noncritical patients and acutely ill patients and patients suspected of infectious disorders. Potentially contagious conditions require equipment that is easily sanitized or disposable. Handheld units are preferred and disposable gel packets are useful in potentially contaminated circumstances. Obtaining a previous or baseline scan is essential for managing the outcome. The optimum initial scan for acute respiratory distress syndrome (ARDS) includes IVC and cardiac sonography. If pulmonary embolus is suspected, evaluation of the deep venous system may be included. Imaging of the lung is clinically divided into outpatient, noncritical patients and acutely ill patients and patients suspected of infectious disorders. Potentially contagious conditions require equipment that is easily sanitized or disposable. Handheld units are preferred and disposable gel pacs are useful in potentially contaminated circumstances. Obtaining a previous or baseline scan is essential for managing the outcome. The optimum initial scan for acute respiratory distress syndrome (ARDS) includes IVC and cardiac sonography. If pulmonary embolus is suspected, evaluation of the deep venous system may be included. Prognostication of severity and mortality risk may be based on a CT scoring system of time from disease progression to resolution and percentage of pulmonary parenchyma involved with Grade 1 less than 5% to Grade 5 more than 75% for the GGO, crazy paving pattern and consolidation. Idiopathic pulmonary fibrosis presents with sub pleural consolidations, nonhomogeneous B-line distribution and areas of frank pulmonary consolidation.

8.15.1 Bedside IVC Imaging

In critical cases where pulmonary emboli is suspected, CT angiography may be performed. As an alternative, ultrasound imaging of the IVC inferior vena cava and right ventricular (RV) volume overload may be utilized at the bedside. The addition of AI artificial intelligence automated cardiac imaging analysis (recently cleared by the FDA and European CE mark authorities) is important since the RV is difficult to evaluate due to its unique structure and location. Regarding Covid-19 mortality, recent studies show a significant link between right heart failure and a Mt. Sinai Medical Center (New York City) study showed 31% of patients hospitalized with Covid-19 had right ventricle failure and 41% of this subset who died had findings of right ventricular dilation or enlargement. Since bedside diagnostics are currently normalized worldwide, it is useful to differentiate acute pulmonary disease from acute heart failure (AHF) during the routine lung ultrasound exploration. Point of care ultrasound (POCUS) of the inferior vena cava (IVC) is accepted as a quick and useful modality for diagnosis and determination of prognosis of patients with AHF. A study of the IVC using IVC expiratory diameter and/or IVC collapsibility index demonstrated a IVC expiratory dimension greater than 2.0 cm and an IVC collapsibility index of less than 30% suggest that acute dyspnea is likely to be due to AHF [48].

8.16   Image Guided Procedures

CT, CT-LUS fusion, and sonography-guided punctures have a low rate of complications. The rate of pneumothorax is 2.8%; 1% require drainage. Hemorrhage or hemoptysis is observed in 0–2%. Data concerning air embolism or even death are not available so far. Tumor dissemination through the procedure of puncture is of little clinical significance and very rare, in less than 0.003% of cases. In cases of malignant pleural mesothelioma, it is slightly more common. When surgery is performed, the site of puncture is also resected.

8.16.1 Pneumothorax After Puncture

If the focus of the procedure is no longer visible after the puncture, the likelihood of a pneumothorax is high. This can be reliably detected by sonography, through the absence of respiration-dependent gliding movement of the pleura. The quantity of free air can only be measured by obtaining a chest radiograph or limited CT scan. A pneumothorax usually reaches its maximum dimensions after 3 h, so the decision regarding a therapeutic procedure is made thereafter, when the pneumothorax is smaller. If the patient is symptomatic or if a larger volume is present, the patient is initially given protracted thoracocentesis. The success rate within the first 10 h is 90%. In the event of renewed collapse, the clinician may use a percutaneous drain and a catheter with a small lumen. A routine chest radiograph or follow-up CT scan is not required after routine CT or sonography-guided puncture.

8.16.2 Pulmonary Fibrosis

As mentioned earlier, survivors are experiencing either new organ system disorders or complications of ventilator dependency and pulmonary fibrosis. CT and ultrasound are useful in the investigation of these disorders and useful in follow up of potentially chronic conditions. While lung CT abnormalities attain greatest severity approximately 10 days after onset of symptoms and tend to reduce after 14 days during the absorption phase with patients achieving normal living ability by about 2 months after onset, CT findings may remain apparent. CT images in the early recovery phase show reduction of GGO and reduced consolidation but pulmonary fibrosis appears as fibrous shadows such as fibrous stripes, subpleural lines and traction bronchiectasis in multiple lung lobes. This finding has been documented previously in SARS patients discharged after treatment. One can follow up fibrosis with nonradiation imaging such as chest wall elastography and diaphragmatic ultrasound to compare with clinical respiratory evaluation [48].

8.16.3 High Resolution Pleural Imaging

In the months following patients with very minimal CT images, the clinical symptoms in some progress due to a chronic fibrotic response even as the imaging findings improve. This makes the pleural findings an important parameter and suggests initial and serial follow-up with noninvasive high resolution 3D ultrasound with elastographic scanning (Fig. 8.28) The normal pleural thickness at 18 MHz linear transducer imaging is 0.3–0.5 mm and the normal pleural echo may be inhomogeneous due to the expected respiratory motion. Similarly, the expected A-lines have the same features. A pathologically thickened pleura line is optimally imaged with a 3D 17 MHz linear probe or 18 MHz convex probe. The diaphragmatic pleural interface is important since most of the pathology is found in this area which has some B-line activity in recumbent positions or in

Fig. 8.28 CT of right upper lobe with very early ground glass opacity (red square). Patient developed increased dyspnea after infiltrate cleared on CT. (Figure courtesy Dr. John Melnick, Lenox Hill Radiology, New York)

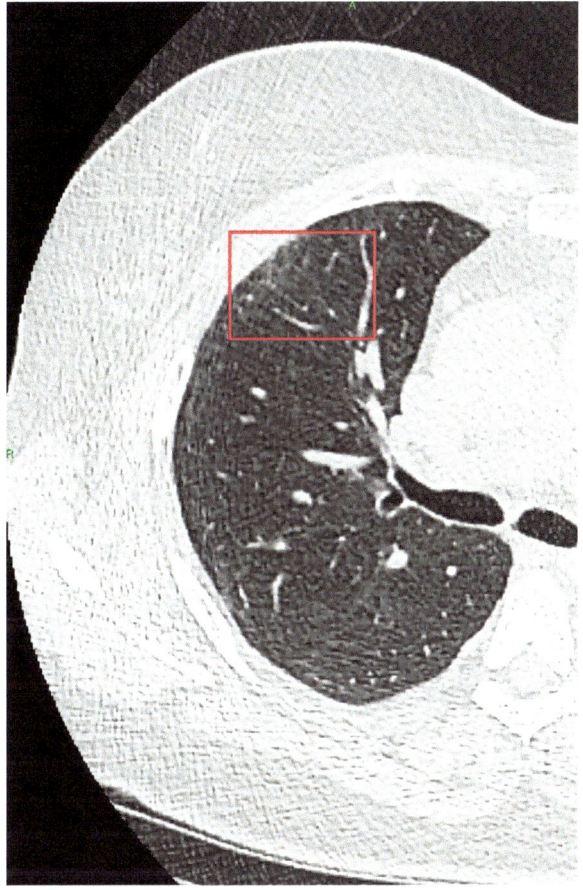

elderly patients so the pleural thickness is helpful in determining disease aggression. A thin pleural line with good respiratory excursion (Fig. 8.29) suggests healthy tissues. Inflammatory or neoplastic hepatic or splenic disorder may cause attenuation through the glands and abnormal findings at the parenchymal-pleural interface (Fig. 8.30).

8.16.4 Tissue Elastography

Tissue density imaged by elastography has been performed on the liver (Fig. 8.31a, b) breast, prostate, thyroid and skin for many years with high accuracy. Desmoplastic tumors and inflammatory fibrosis alter the elastic modulus and are measured on the color-coded side bar. Since the degree of pleural thickening is roughly proportional to the length of recovery, a study may be performed using this technology as a surrogate marker for future treatment assessment. Tissue calcium deposition is observed

Fig. 8.29 Fibrotic liver tissue producing artifactual diaphragmatic pleural outline

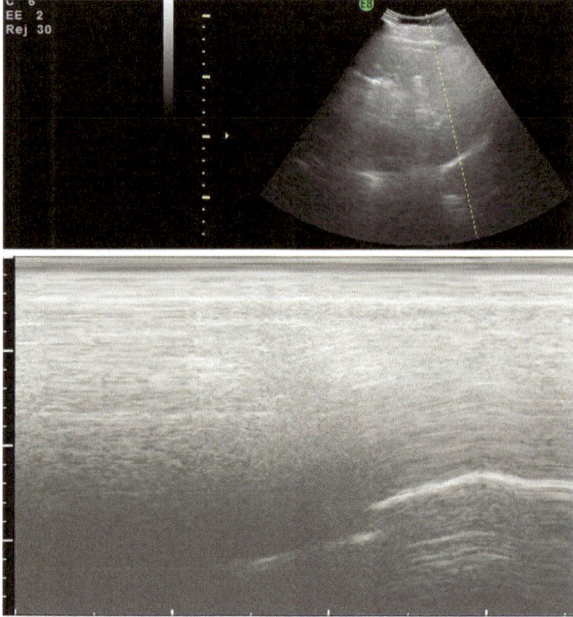

Fig. 8.30 Elastography normal liver with blue soft tissue density of benign tissue

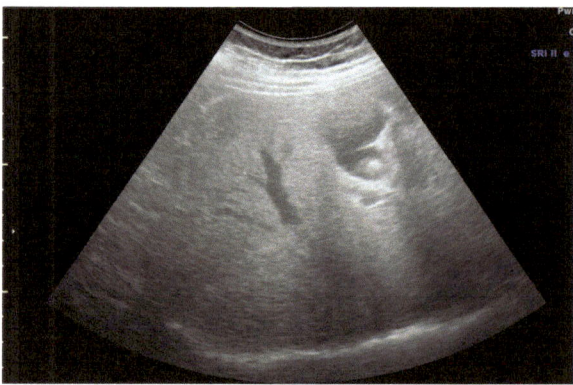

in some malignant processes and chronic inflammatory disorders therefore elastography imaging is combined with ultrasound and radiographic studies.

8.17   Future Directions

8.17.1 Algorithm Advances

Overall, the task of computerized registration for medical image fusion is a non-trivial task which has gained much traction in the computer vision community over the past several decades. Yet it is still very much an unsolved problem, and significant

Fig. 8.31 Elastography breast tumor (left) red indicates high density of malignant tissue

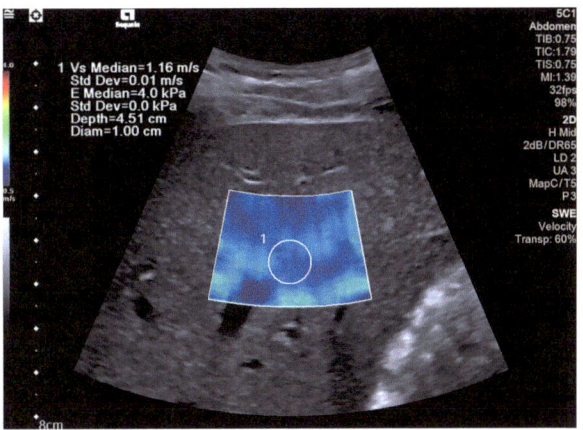

research is still required. The wide range of clinical problems with Covid-19 lung disease supports escalating platforms of technology and algorithms, since stable patients at home require imaging and treatment options different from acutely ill ICU patients. A problem arises when one wishes to (a) evaluate registration accuracy, and (b) decide is an algorithm "good enough." To evaluate registration, one may wish to use manual fiducials identified within the image and evaluate the displacement, determine the overlap of the objects of interest, or determine how well an algorithm performed in a specific task, such as accurately sampling a tumor in the case of MRI TRUS fusion biopsies. In terms of commercial systems, "good enough" may also require consideration of the cost of development, ease of application and the speed of the system. A real-time registration algorithm which has an error of 3 mm may be sufficient to consistently sample a tumor in terms of a biopsy, and may be considered "better" than an algorithm which takes 1 h yet has an error of 1 mm. It truly depends on one's goal for the registration algorithm, and in the future many more fusion systems will likely employ more sophisticated and advanced registration algorithms.

8.17.2 Volumetric Imaging

3D volumetric image reconstruction generates a data set that commonly registers color-coded images useful for histogram analysis in vessel density studies. This same algorithm may be used to map the gray level density in non-Doppler images. The so-called "white lung" appearance of massive B-line aggregation volume may be semi-quantified by measuring the mean gray level which is an indirect representation of the amount of "white" lung or multiple, confluent B-lines. Additional use for noninvasive imaging is documentation of adverse affects of treatment (allergic response) and exposure to the widely used sanitization procedures (toxicity). Allergy has been widely studied with patch testing but this dermal elevation may be examined with high-resolution ultrasound for depth, Doppler ultrasound and confocal microscopy for neovascularity quantitative measurements. Regarding toxicity, the recent massive personal and commercial distribution of recent sanitizing options has not been evaluated for short- and long-term effects on the lung, skin and eyes. This is a future role for advanced imaging technologies for evaluation of new and potentially harmful technologies.

8.17.3 Clinical Testing

- Early risk stratification in Covid-19 remains a laboratory and clinical challenge. A recent Lancet article demonstrated a clear relationship between high viral load and mortality. Transforming qualitative testing into a quantitative measurement of viral load will assist clinicians in risk-stratifying patients but is time consuming and not useful for emergency triage. Using cutaneous imaging ultrasound and optical technologies is real time and may be used for choosing among available therapies and trials. Imaging may become a surrogate marker for viral load used at triage to affect isolation measures on the basis of potential infectivity. Future studies could address SARS-CoV-2 viral load dynamics and the quantitative relationship with neutralizing antibodies, cytokines and quantitative imaging technologies such as 3D/4D Doppler Histogram analysis, reflective confocal microscopy (RCM) and optical computed tomography (OCT) [49].

8.18 Summary

Characteristic Lung US findings in Covid-19 patients: Covid foci are mainly noted in posterior lung fields-often bilaterally. Thickened pleural lines with rare pleural effusions are expected. 3D histogram analysis shows pleural irregularity. Small consolidations are nonlobar and translobar. Decreased blood supply on vascular Doppler imaging in consolidated areas and diminishing regional B-lines suggests clinical improvement. Multimodality imaging encapsulates the use of A-mode, B-mode, 3D and 4D, Doppler, vascular histogram, elastography, micro-optical imaging, image guided fusion and interventional radiologic techniques. Robotic diagnostics and image guided robotic treatment ensure staff protection during procedures and avoid cross contamination of regional facilities and adjacent personnel. Telemedicine options offer at home bedside self-scanning assistance as remote diagnostic service with state of the art ultrasound devices. Underserved regional areas participate in real-time communication with expert radiologists via comprehensive virtual overreading through web-based partnerships.

References

1. Clevert A. Lung ultrasound in patients with Covid-19 disease 2020 AIUM Webinar Series-6/4/20.
2. Volpicelli G, Elbarbary M, Blaivas M, et al. International evidence-based recommendations for point-of-care lung ultrasound. Intensive Care Med. 2012;38:577–91.

3. Koenig SJ, Narasimhan M, Mayo PH. Thoracic ultrasonography for the pulmonary specialist. Chest. 2011;140:1332–41.
4. Lichtenstein DA, Menu Y. A bedside ultrasound sign ruling out pneumothorax in the critically ill: lung sliding. Chest. 1995;108:1345–8.
5. Lichtenstein D, Mezière G, Biderman P, Gepner A. The "lung point": an ultrasound sign specific to pneumothorax. Intensive Care Med. 2000;26:1434–40.
6. Lichtenstein D, Mezière G, Biderman P, Gepner A, Barré O. The comet-tail artifact: an ultrasound sign of alveolar-interstitial syndrome. Am J Respir Crit Care Med. 1997;156:1640–6.
7. Copetti R, Soldati G, Copetti P. Chest sonography: a useful tool to differentiate acute cardiogenic pulmonary edema from acute respiratory distress syndrome. Cardiovasc Ultrasound. 2008;6:16.
8. Agricola E, Bove T, Oppizzi M, et al. "Ultrasound comet-tail images": a marker of pulmonary edema—a comparative study with wedge pressure and extravascular lung water. Chest. 2005;127:1690–5.
9. Lichtenstein DA, Mezière GA, Lagoueyte JF, Biderman P, Goldstein I, Gepner A. A-lines and B-lines: lung ultrasound as a bedside tool for predicting pulmonary artery occlusion pressure in the critically ill. Chest. 2009;136:1014–20.
10. Lichtenstein DA, Mezière GA. Relevance of lung ultrasound in the diagnosis of acute respiratory failure: the BLUE protocol. Chest. 2008;134:117–25.
11. Lichtenstein DA, Lascols N, Mezière G, Gepner A. Ultrasound diagnosis of alveolar consolidation in the critically ill. Intensive Care Med. 2004;30:276–81.
12. Zanobetti M, Poggioni C, Pini R. Can chest ultrasonography substitute standard chest radiography for evaluation of acute dyspnea in the emergency department? Chest. 2011;139:1140–7.
13. Balik M, Plasil P, Waldauf P, Pazout J, Fric M, Otahal M, Pachl J. Ultrasound estimation of volume of pleural fluid in mechanically ventilated patients. Intensive Care Med. 2006;32:318.
14. Remerand F, Dellamonica J, Mao Z, et al. Multiplane ultrasound approach to quantify pleural effusion at the bedside. Intensive Care Med. 2010;36:656–64.
15. Vega JML, Gordo M, Velez S, et al. Pneumomediastinum and spontaneous pneumothorax as an extrapulmonary complication of COVID-19 disease. Emerg Radiol. 2020;3:1–4.
16. Bard RL. Crescent sign in pulmonary hematoma. Respiration. 1975;32:247–51.
17. Bard RL. Crescent sign in pulmonary hematoma. US Air Force Med J. 1970;1:11–3.
18. Bard RL. Pneumomediastinum complicating pregnancy. Respiration. 1975;32:185–8.
19. Soldati G, Smargiassi A, Inchingolo R, et al. Proposal for international standardization for the use of lung ultrasound in Covid-19 patients. J Ultrasound Med. 2020;39(7):1413–9.
20. Boubaker M, Haboussi M, et al. Finite element simulation of interactions between pelvic organs: predictive model of the prostate motion in the context of radiotherapy. J Biomech. 2009;42:1862–8.
21. Brock K, Nichol A, et al. Accuracy and sensitivity of finite element model-based deformable registration of the prostate. Med Phys. 2008;35(9):4019–25.
22. Chappelow J, Bloch BN, et al. Elastic registration of multimodal prostate MRI and histology via multiattribute combined mutual information. Med Phys. 2011;38(4):2005–18.
23. Chi Y, Liang J, Yan D. A material sensitivity study on the accuracy of deformable organ registration using linear biomechanical models. Med Phys. 2006;33(2):421–33.
24. Fei B, Lee Z, et al. Image registration for interventional MRI guided procedures: Interpolation methods, similarity measurements, and applications to the prostate. Biomedical Image Registration. Berlin: Springer; 2003. p. 321–9.
25. Fiard G, Hohn N, et al. Targeted MRI-guided prostate biopsies for the detection of prostate cancer: initial clinical experience with real-time 3-dimensional transrectal ultrasound guidance and magnetic resonance/transrectal ultrasound image fusion. J Urol. 2013;81(6):1372–8.
26. Greene W, Chelikani S, et al. Constrained non-rigid registration for use in image-guided adaptive radiotherapy. Med Image Anal. 2009;13:809–17.
27. Hensel J, Menard C, et al. Development of multiorgan finite element-based prostate deformation model enabling registration of endorectal coil magnetic resonance imaging for radiotherapy planning. Intl J Radiat Oncol Biol Phys. 2007;68(5):1522–8.

28. Holia M, Thaker V. Image registration for recovering affine transformation using Nelder Mead Simplex method for optimization. Intl J Image Process. 2009;3(5):218–29.
29. Maes F, Collignon A, et al. Multimodality image registration by maximization of mutual information. IEEE Trans Med Imaging. 1997;16(2):187–98.
30. Maintz JBA, Viergever MA. A survey of medical image registration. Med Image Anal. 1998;2(1):1–36.
31. Marks L, Young S, Natarajan S. MRI-ultrasound fusion or guidance of targeted prostate biopsy. Curr Opin Urol. 2013;23(1):43–50.
32. Mitra J, Martí R, et al. Prostate multimodality image registration based on B-splines and quadrature local energy. Int J Comput Assist Radiol Surg. 2012;7(3):445–54.
33. Natarajan S, Marks LS, et al. Clinical application of a 3D ultrasound-guided prostate biopsy system. Urol Oncol Semin Orig Investig. 2011;29(3):334–42.
34. Ogura S, Tokuda J, et al. MRI signal intensity based B-spline nonrigid registration for pre- and intraoperative imaging during prostate brachytherapy. J Mag Reson Imag. 2009;30(5):1052–8.
35. Pinto P, Chung PH, et al. Magnetic resonance imaging/ultrasound fusion guided prostate biopsy improves cancer detection following transrectal ultrasound biopsy and correlates with multiparametric magnetic resonance imaging. J Urol. 2011;186(4):1281–5.
36. Rais-Bahrami S, Siddiqui M, et al. Utility of multiparametric MRI suspicion levels in detecting prostate cancer. J Urol. 2013;190(5):1721–7. https://doi.org/10.1016/j.uro.2013.05.052.
37. Rastinehad A, Baccala AA, et al. D'Amico risk stratification correlates with degree of suspicion of prostate cancer on multiparametric magnetic resonance imaging. J Urol. 2011;185(3):815–20.
38. Salvi J, Matabosch C, et al. A review of recent range image registration methods with accuracy evaluation. Image Vis Comput. 2007;25(5):578–96.
39. Sonn GA, Chang E, et al. Value of targeted prostate biopsy using magnetic resonance–ultrasound fusion in men with prior negative biopsy and elevated prostate-specific antigen. Euro Urol. 2014;65(4):809–15. https://doi.org/10.1016/j.eururo.2013.03.025.
40. Turkbey P, Choyke PL. Multiparametric MRI and prostate cancer diagnosis and risk stratification. Curr Opin Urol. 2012;22(4):310–5.
41. Ukimura O, Desai MM, et al. 3-dimensional elastic registration system of prostate biopsy location by real-time 3-dimensional transrectal ultrasound guidance with magnetic resonance/ transrectal ultrasound image fusion. J Urol. 2012;187(3):1080–6.
42. Viola P, Wells WM III. Alignment by maximization of mutual information. Int J Comput Vision. 1997;24(2):137–54.
43. Wachowiak M, Smolikova R, et al. An approach to multimodal biomedical image registration utilizing particle swarm optimization. IEEE Trans Evol Comput. 2004;8(3):289–301.
44. Wells W III, Viola P, et al. Multi-modal volume registration by maximization of mutual information. Med Image Anal. 1996;1(1):35–51.
45. Xu S, Kruecker J, et al. Real-time MRI-TRUS fusion for guidance of targeted prostate biopsies. Comput Aided Surg. 2008;13(5):255–64.
46. Zhang B, Arola DD, et al. Three-dimensional elastic image registration based on strain energy minimization: application to prostate magnetic resonance imaging. J Digital Imag. 2011;24(4):573–85.
47. Zogal P, Sakas E, et al. BiopSee®—transperineal stereotactic navigated prostate biopsy. J Contemp Brachy. 2011;3(2):91–5.
48. DARWISH O, Mahani A, Kataria S, et al. Diagnosis of acute heart failure using inferior vena cava ultrasound. J Ultrasound Med. 2020;39:1367–78.
49. Pujadas E, Chaudry F, McBride R, et al. Sars-CoV-2 virl load predicts mortality. Lancet. 2020;8(9):22–6. https://doi.org/10.1016/S2213-2600(20)30354-4.

Respiratory Dynamics: Function and Breath Management

Linda Carroll

9.1 Introduction

Oral communication requires a coordination of respiratory function, laryngeal function, and resonance/articulatory function. Therefore, compromise of respiratory function directly impacts overall health as well as the ability to communicate needs/wants and actively participate in society. Good respiratory function is also essential for overall systemic health, transporting oxygen to the blood stream, helping maintain adequate circulation for physical and cognitive demands.

There are three main body types—ectomorph, mesomorph, endomorph—with each utilizing slightly different respiratory kinematics. Somatotypes were developed by William Sheldon in the 1940s, and have remained a focus research area in respiration and breath management. Ectomorphs have high relative linearity features, mesomorphs have high relative musculoskeletal features, and endomorphs have high relative fatness. Anecdotal reports include lower breathing patterns and potential for some paradoxic movements among endomorphs, while mesomorphs and ectomorphs tend to involve more rib cage expansion during stronger breath demands. Chatterjee et al. [1] did find significant influence of body type for available lung capacity, with endomorphs having poorest lung capacity. This may become an important factor when developing treatment plans for individuals with respiratory deficits.

During inhalation, the breath volume for all body types depends on the intended task. Tidal breathing is approximately 400–500 mL (or 7 mL/kg) for an adult, with adjustments for sex, age, height and overall health. During heavy exercise and/or projected voice demands (speaking or singing), increased respiratory volumes are

L. Carroll (✉)
The Children's Hospital of Philadelphia, Philadelphia, PA, USA

Department of Communication Sciences and Disorders, University of New Hampshire, Durham, NH, USA

© The Author(s), under exclusive license to Springer Nature Switzerland AG 2021
R. L. Bard (ed.), *Image-Guided Management of COVID-19 Lung Disease*,
https://doi.org/10.1007/978-3-030-66614-9_9

required. Vital capacity in adults is greater for males (4500 mL) than females (~3500 mL) and affected age, height and sex. Vital capacity is determined by the sum of inspiratory reserve volume, tidal volume, and expiratory reserve volume, as measured by spirometry. Other respiratory measures of importance include minute ventilation, or the volume of gas exchange per minute, which is affected by physical conditioning and exercise demand.

Inhalation begins with contraction of the diaphragm and expansion of the thoracic cavity (vertical, anteroposterior, and transverse), with a pressure change occurring in accordance with Boyle's Law. Exhalation is a passive event, but more active contraction of the expiratory muscles is employed for many tasks such as louder speech and singing. During respiration, the air flows from regions of higher pressure to regions of lower pressure. Because of pleural linkage, an increase in thoracic volume stretches the lungs, expands the alveolar air, and causes a decrease in alveolar pressure.

During normal respiration, air flow is mostly laminar, but disease states can cause air flow to be predominately turbulent. During a disease state, there are changes in manner and number of breaths per minute, and changes in breath volume, which affect respiration for life purposes and phonation purposes. Increased respiratory effort has been reported to increase with higher demands on expiration and inspiration [2, 3]. Unless performing whole body exercise at a very high intensity, chronic changes in respiratory function or a perception of dyspnea does not occur even with repeated respiratory challenges in normal subjects [4–6].

From a respiratory standpoint, phonation requires a steady pressure head against the vocal folds. In addition, respiratory drive must be strong enough to protect the airway from foreign bodies. When respiratory skills, or respiratory control, inhibit the ability to access inhalation and exhalation on demand, phonation and protection of the airway becomes challenged and patients can become fearful.

9.2   Impact of Diseases on Respiratory Function

There are a myriad of diseases and conditions that can affect respiratory function. This chapter addresses a subset of the more frequent or concerning diagnoses. The impact on function and communication is included for each diagnosis.

Asthma is a chronic inflammation and narrowing of the airways, and may begin in childhood or may arise due to exercise. Impact of asthma includes restrictions for some physical activities. Symptoms include chest tightness, difficult access inhalation, presence of wheezing and coughing. Severe attacks can be fatal, and patients with asthma need to have a rescue inhaler or bronchodilator available to soothe the constricted bronchi and re-establish easy airway. Although breathing exercises may be helpful, it is essential that medical management be present. Fluticasone can improve ease of breathing but does have some risk of accompanying dysphonia and/ or yeast infection [7]. Other oral medications can be helpful, and patients should always discuss their voice vs. respiratory needs with their pulmonologist prior to, and during use of, any asthma medication. When an inhaler is used, it is important for patients to rinse with mouth/posterior oropharynx to remove any irritant from the propellant (this can lower the risk for yeast infection). Diagnosis of asthma may be confirmed through pulmonary function testing (PFT), examining control of exhalation and inhalation. It is important to note that PFT and bronchodilators can be used to determine if dyspnea is due to asthma or laryngospasm. PFT has a flattened inspiratory loop for laryngospasm, but not for asthma. In addition, asthma patients experience improved lung function with bronchodilators, but this is not always the case for patients with laryngospasm. Due to difficulty with inhalation, patients with asthma (and with laryngospasm) typically experience inability to access voice to call for help and often rely on nonverbal communication to request help.

Allergies create inflammation and changes in secretion balance in the all phonatory subsystems. While nasal congestion can affect ability to project the voice, and laryngeal inflammation can limit ability to achieve normal voicing features, the respiratory impact undermines ease of phonation and non-phonatory tasks. Diagnosis of allergies varies depending on whether the allergy is to a food item or environmental irritant. Food allergies may be identified through skin test, known response to ingestion of a particular food, or through visible reactions (such as rash, hives, etc.). While allergy shots may desensitize environmental allergies, food allergies are managed by avoidance of exposure until there is strong suspicion for safe ingestion of that food items. Environmental allergies (seasonal allergies) are common and can create difficulty with respiration, phonation, resonance, and can cause eye irritation and increase risk for chronic rhinosinusitis. Allergy sensitivity may change over the years, but many allergies present prepuberty, or any allergies to drugs often stay for a lifetime. Medical management (for environmental allergies) and use of nasal wash can dramatically improve the patient's quality of life. Individuals with food allergies may have severe compromise, including anaphylaxis. Food allergies require ready access to an Epi-pen or Benadryl to rapidly reduce the risk of airway closure. It is important to note that continuous breathing resistance exercises may be quite beneficial while awaiting response to medical management. With allergies affecting access to resonance, humming on "n" with use of pitch change can help break up some congestion. Seasonal allergies affect clarity of speech, voice quality, ease of breathing, and may increase risk for development of phonotraumatic lesions (due to imbalance of the subsystems of phonation and resonance/articulation).

Bronchitis and *Pneumonia* affect the health of one or both lungs, and is marked with elevated fever, chronic coughing (particularly if longer than 3 weeks), shortness of breath, rapid breath patterns, and generalized fatigue. These infections of the lungs may be viral or bacterial. Risk factors for both bronchitis and pneumonia include viral exposure, exposure to air pollution, and/or a history of smoking or chronic disease (asthma, COPD, heart disease), as well as age (younger than age 2 years, or older than 65 years). Diagnosis can be confirmed with chest X-ray, pulse oximetry, sputum test, or through auditory sounds (cracking or bubbling) heard with a stethoscope. Due to difficulty with accessing breath, patients may find themselves confined to bedrest, and often have difficulty avoiding coughing throughout the day and night. The impact of fever further affects low energy, and triggers difficulty with activities of daily living. Following pneumonia, it is important for the patient to use inhalation and exhalation respiratory exercises to re-establish adequate breath management for functional activities. While it is traditional for patients to use an incentive spirometer and other exercises to help inhalation strength and volume post-pneumonia, it is equally important to re-establish strength and endurance of exhalation and breath support. Expiratory exercises include repeated /pʰ/ and /м/ exercises, as well as prolonged stable exhalation with pursed lips. For professional voice users, it may take 4–6 months to recover normal and comfortable access to those respiratory demands following pneumonia. Patients with bronchitis typically need greater attention on control of chronic cough.

The *COVID-19* pandemic suddenly alerted the general public on the risks of pulmonary compromise and the rapid demise of health. The inflammatory process of COVID-19 can gradually accumulate, often affecting the respiratory system first, with the impending severity not noticed by many patients in the early stages of infection. Severe cases of COVID-19 can lead to Acute Respiratory Distress Syndrome [8]. Gradual changes in lung volume are easily measured with pulse oximetry, but prior to COVID-19, few individuals routinely measured their oxygenation levels when feeling "slightly under the weather." Due to changes in the lung epithelium from COVID-19 infection [9], the bronchi and bronchioles have difficulty transporting air and the necessary rapid diffusion of oxygen and carbon dioxide through the walls of the squamous epithelium of the alveolar ducts and alveoli. The inflammation of the lung tissue creates progressive compromise of breathing, which attributes to the patient awareness of decline of oxygen control. The compromise of oxygenation (hypoxemia) can be easily measured using pulse oximetry. A simple pulse oximeter device may be used by subjects at home, allowing them to determine if an underlying infection affecting the lungs may be present. If pulse oximetry is less than 90%, medical assessment is *essential.* Dysphonia has been found in 27% of patients with mild to moderate COVID-19, with greater risk for females. Severity of dyspnea, dysphagia, ear pain, face pain, throat pain and nasal obstruction was higher in the dysphonic COVID-19 group compared with non-dysphonic group [10].

Following COVID-19, patients need to follow many of the same respiratory exercise program commonly used with patients who have had pneumonia. Use of resistance breathing exercises (see Appendix 1) is essential for patients with known or suspected COVID-19. With frequent use of inhalation and exhalation resistance, the patient can strengthen access to breath control. Some patients with confirmed COVID-19 have anecdotally reported ability to avoid use of a respirator with hourly resistance breathing exercises. Research is warranted to determine the extent of improvement with self-exercise however due to the severity of respiratory distress with COVID-19. There is increasing evidence for risk of long-term effects from COVID-19 for the lungs (scarring) as well as circulatory, renal, hepatic, and hematological systems [11]. Any patient who has a history of COVID-19 should be monitored with greater attention to respiratory, circulatory and inflammatory changes.

Chronic Obstructive Pulmonary Disease (COPD) has a common etiology of emphysema and chronic bronchitis, but may also be related to alpha-1-antitrypsin

(AAt) deficiency. COPD is more common at age 40+. Smoking and long-term exposure to gases or particulate matter are the highest risk factors. Hardin and Silverman [12] did report females to have a higher genetic risk. COPD results in difficulty accessing adequate breath for speech and exercise. Patients may also report chest tightness, wheezing, stridor and coughing. Because COPD is a long-term illness, patients experience permanent changes and limitation in functional activities, and remain at higher risk for other diseases. Speech may be labored in COPD patients due to poor respiratory function.

Collagen vascular disease has been found to affect respiratory function in children, with most common effect of pulmonary restriction, and may also be present for adults with collagen disease [13]. Limited research is present, but suggests the need to investigate collagen disease when vital capacity is less than 80% of predicted and to ensure that idiopathic interstitial pneumonia is not due to underlying collagen vascular disease [14, 15]. Medical/surgical management is essential.

Mixed connective tissue disease (MCTD) is known to affect respiration, and early detection (particularly in children) improves the ability to design targeted therapies to reduce overall morbidity and mortality [16]. Individuals diagnosed with chronic heart failure are at greater risk for restricted respiration, which is visible in pulmonary function testing [17]. There is some evidence that lung function can serve as a differential diagnosis for various connective tissue diseases [18]. Team management of cardiac and respiratory is needed for these patients.

Polymyositis/dermatomyositis (PM-DM) is an inflammatory disease of muscle and skin causing muscle weakness. PM-DM can increase risk for pneumonia, similar to other autoimmune disease, and these patients may suffer more severe infection and slower recovery rates [19]. PM-DM can lead to respiratory failure, aspiration and dysphagia, and can cause cardiac complications [20, 21]. Ji et al. [22] found patients with a fever tended to have a higher frequency of PM-DM associated Interstitial lung disease.

Pregnancy impacts ease of breath control in the third trimester as the fetus expands and limits lung expansion for inhalation and contraction of abdominal-diaphragmatic support for phonation, rather than only for support of the fetus (and fetal movements). As the fetus grows, at-rest breath control becomes shallower and projected voice use becomes more difficult. While respiration may be more effortful, pregnant women are able to access both speech and singing right up to labor contractions. Following delivery of the newborn, patients are typically recommended to rest for 7–10 days before returning to respiratory and physical activities, gradually increasing to their pre-pregnancy routine.

Rheumatoid arthritis (RA) commonly affects the laryngeal structures and is also recognized to trigger inflammation in the lungs which may lead to scarring. RA primarily affects joints (especially synovial joints), but can lead to long-term inflammation and interstitial lung disease). RA contributes to shortness of breath, chronic dry cough, fatigue, weakness and loss of appetite [23]. Environmental and occupational factors, particularly exposure to dust and/or tobacco smoke, has been found to increase risk for RA [24, 25]. This questions the relationship between mucosal irritation and inflammation of the joints. RA is more common in women, and is more likely to be diagnosed due to voice or swallow changes due to laryngeal involvement. Patients with RA may report globus sensation, hoarseness, dyspnea, stridor, dysphagia, odynophonia, and/or odynophagia. Laryngeal findings include ankylosis of the cricoarytenoid joint, arytenoid erythema, and rheumatoid nodules ("Bamboo nodes") on vocal folds. There is no cure for RA, and patients with RA report frustration with sudden exacerbation of symptoms despite medical management. While vocal and respiratory range-of-motion exercises may help access to respiratory and laryngeal demands for oral communication, medical management and lifestyle accommodations are considered the primary management for RA.

Sarcoidosis is a multisystem autoimmune system disease, more common in females aged 20–40 years and more common in African-Americans. When sarcoidosis is present in the lungs, there is a persistent cough with shortness of breath, wheezing and chest pain. There is no cure, but medical management can be helpful. In severe cases, organ transplant may be considered. While breathing resistance exercises and physical range-of-motion exercises may produce short-term benefits, the chief limitation of inflammation across organs is not easily managed and directly impacts access to projected voice and activities of daily living. Sarcoidosis typically triggers effortful breathing and phonation, and inflammation may cause reduced labial movements for clear speech.

Sclerosis is an autoimmune disease causing skin thickening from excessive collagen production, with fibrosis, blood vessel disease, and inflammation. This disease is more common among younger males of African-American ethnicity [26]. The vast majority of scleroderma patients exhibit abnormal pulmonary function testing. Sclerosis may affect numerous organs, but direct involvement of interstitial lung disease (ILD) and pulmonary hypertension (PH) is the leading cause of death for these patients [27]. Patients with scleroderma are more susceptible to respiratory/pulmonary infections and this contributes to morbidity and excess mortality [28]. Because of difficulty accessing easy breath management as well as common laryngeal findings (inflammation of vocal fold mucosa, submucosal nodules), sclerosis patients may present with hoarse voice with reduced projection and endurance. Reduced access to normal respiratory function causes shortened communication phrases, and a sense of breathlessness. Medical/surgical management is essential in these patients, but respiratory and physical exercises can improve some access to better respiratory skills.

Sjögren's syndrome causes dryness of the oral cavity, larynx and eyes, but can also trigger interstitial lung disease and overall joint pain. Sjögren's is a common chronic systemic autoimmune disease that affects the exocrine glands necessary for healthy tissue. Patients commonly complain of a dry cough, hoarseness, and dry eyes. Pulmonary involvement may not be a common initial feature of this disease, but is common in later stages, and can be a cause of death [29]. Lung involvement is an important prognostic indicator in Sjögren's. Medications are the common management for sicca affecting the mouth, larynx and eyes, but there is hope in the future for gene therapy [30]. Dysphonia and vocal fatigue associated with laryngeal sicca may be reduced with vocal range-of-motion exercises (improved prosody), but lubrication of the tissues remains a key component to successful management.

Systemic lupus erythematosus (SLE) is more common in women of child-bearing age and is a chronic autoimmune disorder that may affect several organs. Patients typically report symptoms of arthritis, fever, malaise, and a "butterfly" facial rash, and have hoarseness, throat pain, and dyspnea. Patients characteristically experience periods of remission and relapse. When the disease is active, hyperactivity of immune system triggers inflammation, damage to joints, skin, blood, and organs (kidneys, heart, lungs). Nielepkowicz-Gozdzinska et al. [31] found a significant difference in the concentration of interleukin-8 (IL-8) for SLE patients compared to healthy control subjects, as well as lower lung capacity in SLE patients due to pulmonary fibrosis. Management includes immunomodulators (hydroxychloroquine and vitamin D), immunosuppressants, avoidance of ultraviolet light, prevention of comorbidities, as well as general recommendations on sun protection, diet and nutrition, smoking cessation, exercise and appropriate immunization [32, 33]

9.3 Probes for Respiratory Function

9.3.1 Medical Assessment

The gold standard for medical assessment is pulmonary function testing (PFT). A spirometer permits measurement or Forced Vital Capacity (FVC) and Forced Expiratory Volume in the first second of exhalation (FEV1) which serve as critical measures of respiratory function. Reduced FVC is an indicator of pulmonary compromise, loss of lung plasticity, and risk to other organs. Reduced FEV1 suggests the patient may have difficulty generating sufficient aerodynamic drive to protect the airway with cough reflex. Flow volume measures require a pneumotachometer which can then determine the lung volumes and capacities during exhalation and inhalation. When more information on mechanics of speech respiration are needed, more elaborate instrumentation such as volume-pressure body plethysmography, body-surface measurements, and strain gauge measures may be indicated. Spirometry and Flow Volume measurements assist with assessment of respiratory diseases, response to respiratory treatments/therapy, and can serve as baseline measures for employment examinations. These tests are simple to perform, but the equipment does require regular calibration, cleaning/disinfection, and training for the examiner to accurately instruct the subject during the pulmonary testing.

Objective respiratory measures compare observed values against predicted values during the exhalation portion of pulmonary function testing. When %predicted falls below 90%, it may warrant further investigation. If the midflow 50% (forced expiratory flow from 25% to 75% of the exhalation) falls below 80%, there is concern for underling respiratory disease (COPD) or compromise of respiratory function (asthma, allergy, recent bronchitis or pneumonia). A flattened inspiratory loop is strongly suggestive of a laryngospasm, where the vocal folds fail to remain abducted during sudden inhalation.

Aerodynamic measures are valuable to determine efficiency of conversion of respiration to phonation. These measures are common in a speech laboratory and allow measurement of subglottal pressure, transglottal flow, and phonation threshold pressure. Reduced subglottal pressure may signal vocal fold weakness. Increased transglottal flow is a strong indicator of vocal fold insufficiency (common with vocal fold paralysis or presbyphonia). Variable transglottal flow (during sustained vowel) suggests loss of steady pressure head (necessary for speech) and also questions the ability to generate a strong, protective cough. Elevated phonation threshold pressure is consistent with vocal fold stiffness and/or vocal fold mass. Although maximum phonation time (MPT) does yield some information, a reduced MPT may be due to inadequate breath support or laryngeal status. In contrast, exceedingly longer MPT signals laryngeal hyperfunction. It is important to determine if deficits are due to the respiratory component (lungs) or source subsystem (larynx).

9.3.2 Clinical Assessment

There are some clinical observations however, that can lead the clinician and the patient to determine the need for formal testing of respiratory measures. Some observations may be tracked by the patient, while others need skills by a trained professional.

During calm, slow breathing through the nose (for both inhalation and exhalation), adults who are seated typically use 6–8 breaths/min. Breath rates may increase for oral breathing patterns, but a breathing rate of greater than 15 breaths/min and a report of shortness of breath warrants investigation. It is not uncommon for patients to report dyspnea when they have more than 15 breaths/min using nasal breathing, and/or breathing patterns that are more clavicular or thoracic rather than abdominal-diaphragmatic. Interestingly, singing activities have been noted to make many patients feel "better." This may be due to the typical length of sung phrases, which coaxes the subject into 6–12 breaths/min.

During nasal inhalation, there is increased resistance to the airflow at the filter (resonance/articulation) subsystem, which then triggers reduced resistance to airflow at the source (laryngeal) subsystem, which then triggers an increased resistance to the airflow in the lower portions of the lung cavity. Understanding the change in resistance during inhalation/exhalation can improve breathing skill, as well as improving vocal clarity. The subsystems of power, source, and filter work together, compensating and balancing the workload.

Use of aerodynamic resistance exercises (see Appendix 1) can be invaluable when a patient senses sudden laryngeal closure (laryngospasm, anaphylaxis) or when significant shortness of breath arises. Increased resistance during both inhalation and exhalation will reduce laryngeal tension and permit the air to move rather than be trapped. Aerodynamic resistance is easily accomplished for many patients during nasal breathing, but can also be achieved with deflection of the airflow during oral inhalation. Deflection may be achieved through use of a cupped hand, finger(s) against the lips, pursed lips, or articulatory postures (such as "f" or "s" posture). Use of aerodynamic resistance within the oral cavity can be particularly helpful to stop a laryngospasm, or to protect against a sudden odor or airborne debris. Aerodynamic resistance exercises can also strengthen pulmonary drive and respiratory control.

Use of the aerodynamic resistance and use of improved balance of posture can orient the patient to sensing the lower breath patterns. This can be invaluable for patients experiencing dyspnea due to respiratory deficits. Posture, however, remains the most contributor to poor breathing patterns.

When the shoulder blades are balanced in a narrower position, the sternum and upper thoracic cavity do not compress downward, and the floating ribs are more dynamic, allowing for easier breathing. Alexander training [34] focuses on balanced posture of the upper and lower torso for both standing and sitting, and can be beneficial for those patients who have difficulty finding a balanced upper torso posture to improve access to abdominal-diaphragmatic breathing patterns. Patients who have sedentary lifestyle patterns throughout their day, or those who spend a great deal of time focusing on computer monitors need improved monitoring of their upper body tensions. Use of simple physical stretches (Appendix 2) focused on upper torso range-of-motion during the day can improve ease of access to good breath management, allowing the "floating ribs" to strengthen. There should be no appreciable movement of the shoulders during inhalation or exhalation, but you should see (or sense) rib cage expansion and compression.

During inhalation, there should be no audible breath noises (stridor). Audible stridor suggests the need to rule out obstruction and/or glottic flaccidity.

During exhalation, there should be adequate conversion of respiration to phonation to permit speaking the numbers 1–20 on one breath when using a fairly rapid rate of speech. Similarly, adults should be able to sustain "ah" at a comfortable pitch and loudness level for a minimum of 15 s. Deficits in either of these probes suggest the need for laryngeal examination, and to rule out glottic incompetence from vocal fold immobility or a vocal fold mass.

Any sudden change in respiratory skill, phonatory skill, or access to resonance warrants medical evaluation. Likewise, increased effort in access to any subsystem is of concern, whether sudden or gradual. Through responsible self-monitoring of function on the part of the individual, and regular annual medical assessments, respiratory skills vital for multisystem health and adequate access to functional communication can be achieved and maintained throughout the lifespan.

9.4   Exercises to Optimize Breath Management

Physical stretches are typically the first series of exercises to improve breath control, and allow the individual to explore an improved respiratory pattern. Physical exercises may encourage respiration to be more clavicular or thoracic, but optimum speech and singing requires abdominal-diaphragmatic breathing patterns. Some occupations (Broadway performers) require the individual to be able to quickly change from dynamic physical tasks (dancing, choreography) to delicate subsystem coordination for singing and speaking. This requires a rapid reset of breathing patterns, but the amount of rib cage vs. abdominal excursion does vary by body type [35]. Physical stretches gently explore range-of-motion (ROM) of the upper torso, allowing the individual to find the balance for their specific body type.

Respiratory drive and access to quick inhalation and exhalation can be explored with panting exercises. The simple /p/–50 panting exercise tasks the individual with a single unvoiced "p" (/pʰ/) with a small inhalation prior to each "p," with 50 repetitions. Following the initial warm-up of 50 quick pursed exhalations, the exercise goes immediately into a "p"–"la" sequence for 45 s, with the unvoiced strong "p" preceding a random pitched moderately soft, short in duration, sung "la," incorporating the full vocal range (chest voice to falsetto). This exercise requires a fair degree of coordination with the strong unvoiced "p" and then a moderately soft sung "la."

A more elaborate and lengthy exercise is the DEVT Panting exercise, [36] where the individual sings a short vowel (/i,e,a,o,u/) followed by 3 exhale/inhale pantings and continues through a series of other vowels before singing a 5-note ascending-descending scale using staccato, legato and marcato patterns. The DEVT panting exercise requires dynamic respiratory exchange (exhale, inhale) surrounding delicate phonation control patterns.

Vibration therapy (Lip flutters, tongue trills, Lax Vox, Straw phonation) has been used for decades to improve subsystem coordination and balance resistive forces, particularly during voicing. Many of these exercises can be adapted to target only the respiratory system however. Lip flutters (a.k.a. tongue trills or "raspberries") and tongue trills (the rolled "r") may be done unvoiced, using only respiratory drive. With change of loudness in an unvoiced manner, breath support is strengthened.

Lax Vox (water-resistance therapy) and straw phonation may also be performed in an unvoiced manner [37, 38]. Both Lax Vox and Straw phonation use a straw to extend the vocal tract, causing the individual to use increased breath support. Most patients start with a 5 mm straw (children use a smaller diameter straw, and shorter length straw) and adapt to the size that creates the best respiratory drive and subsystem coordination. During Lax Vox, the straw is immersed into water (typically 5 cm water depth immersion), which causes the patient to use stronger respiratory drive, and the straw diameter limits the amount of air flow, as the "bubbles" are sustained over a period of several minutes. Anecdotally, it is important to avoid straw exercises in patients with micrognathia since they often extend the mandible to hold the straw in the bilabial position, causing muscle tension. Most patients however find marked improvement in voice quality and awareness of breath support throughout the vocal range with use of straw exercises.

9.5 Summary

Respiratory skill forms the basis for overall health as well as the ability to communicate needs and wants. Deficits in access to necessary respiration may arise from disease states, posture changes, or deconditioning following a medical event. Respiratory volumes are influenced by age, sex, height, and body type. Monitoring of respiratory function may be a vital indicator for prognosis in a disease state.

While use of some respiratory exercises can help individuals with dyspnea, medical evaluation and care is vital, and team management is often essential for best outcomes.

Appendix 1: Aerodynamic Resistance Exercises

These exercises can be performed while sitting or standing.

Breathe in/out, slowly, trying to use 5–10 beats for inhalation and 5–10 beats for exhalation, with 2 cycles during each probe. You should sense the breath being driven low into the lung cavity. Avoid "starving" yourself for the breath, but seek to trust the breath as it fills and empties the lungs. Observe the sensations in the side ribs and lower ribs, as well as the sensation in the larynx.

Posture 1: cupped hand over mouth and nose (fingers tightly together, creating firm seal over mouth and nose).

Posture 2: pursed lips with three fingers (held together) occluding the lips.

Posture 3: pursed lips with two fingers (held together) occluding the lips (fake cigarette position).

Posture 4: pursed lips with one finger occluding the lips.

Posture 5: pursed, puckered lips (similar to sipping a thick shake or sucking spaghetti).

Posture 6: "f" position (upper teeth contacting lower lip).

Posture 7: tongue tip up behind upper front teeth, mouth fairly closed ("seething" position).

Determine the two posture resistance strategies that work the best for you each day. Use those two postures every 2–3 h, using five breath cycles for each posture.

Note: If you have a diagnosis of laryngospasm, do *not* pause at the end of the exhalation. If you have a diagnosis of chronic cough, do *not* pause at the top of the inhalation.

Appendix 2: Physical Stretches: Perform While Standing

1. Arching: Extend right arm and arc to opposite side (right arm extended, leaning over left shoulder, with body bent toward the left), and take a slow breath to maximally expand the right rib cage. Repeat, taking two breath inhalations with each arc position. Then change to opposite arc, expanding the left rib cage. Repeat sequence three to four times.
2. Hangman: With arms extended and forearms at right angles (like a hangman), inhale and try to maximally expand movement in the front upper chest. Exhale as you bring forearms together in front of you, letting upper chest cave in a bit. Repeat 4×, then relax the shoulder joints. Now, reverse the inhale/exhale posture. With forearms together in front (bend slightly forward so that your back will be slightly rounded), take a breath and maximally expand upper back region. Exhale

as you bring your arms outward and open upper chest forward (like a hangman). Repeat 4 times.

3. Ragdoll: Place hands at waist, thumbs forward and fingers touching posterior rib region, and bend over. Take a slow full breath, driving the breath into your hands (not up your back), and then hold the full inhalation for a few beats. Exhale and feel the ribs come inward. Repeat. When breath expansion feels secure in that position, while holding the breath at full inhalation, change posture to one that is closer to regular standing position. Exhale and repeat. Continue until standing upright. Take breath while standing straight, still feeling lower posterior rib expansion with breath.

4. Discus Gumby: Twist to the left, extending arms behind you: inhale. Sense the transverse and lateral expansion. Repeat. Twist to the right, extending arms behind you: inhale. Repeat. Repeat sequence 3 – 4 times.

5. Figure 8s: Place fists on shoulders, elbows forward; using elbows as "paint-brush," trace the number "8" high, wide and high/low, with 4 tracings clockwise, and 4 tracings counter-clockwise. Then stand, place hand at waist thumbs forward, and sense expansion into your hands.

References

1. Chatterjee P, Bandyopadhyay A, Chatterjee P, Nandy P. Assessment and comparative analysis of different lung capacities in trained athletes according to somatotype. Am J Sports Sci. 2019;7(2):72–7. https://doi.org/10.11648/j.ajss.20190702.14.
2. Supinski GS, Clary SJ, Bark H, Kelsen SG. Effect of inspiratory muscle fatigue on perception of effort during loaded breathing. J Appl Physiol. 1987;62(1):300–7. https://doi.org/10.1152/japp.1987.62.1.300.
3. Suzuki S, Suzuki J, Ishii T, Akahori T, Okubo T. Relationship of respiratory effort sensation to expiratory muscle fatigue during expiratory threshold loading. Am Rev Respir Dis. 1992;145(2 Pt 1):461–6. https://doi.org/10.1164/ajrccm/145.2_Pt_1.461.
4. Tiller NB, Turner LA, Taylor BJ. Pulmonary and respiratory muscle function in response to 10 marathons in 10 days. Eur J Appl Physiol. 2019;119(2):509–18. https://doi.org/10.1007/s00421-018-4037-2.
5. Dempsey JA, Babcock MA. An integrative view of limitations to muscular performance. Adv Exp Med Biol. 1995;384:393–9. https://doi.org/10.1007/978-1-4899-1016-5_31.
6. McKenzie DK, Bellemare F. Respiratory muscle fatigue. Adv Exp Med Biol. 1995;384:401–14. https://doi.org/10.1007/978-1-4899-1016-5_32.
7. DelGaudio JM. Steroid inhaler laryngitis: dysphonia caused by inhaled fluticasone therapy. Arch Otolaryngol Head Neck Surg. 2002;128(6):677–81. https://doi.org/10.1001/archotol.128.6.677.
8. Li X, Ma X. Acute respiratory failure in COVID-19: is it "typical" ARDS? Crit Care. 2020;24(1):198. https://doi.org/10.1186/s13054-020-02911-9.
9. Pérez CA. Looking ahead: the risk of neurologic complications due to COVID-19. Neurol Clin Pract. 2020;10(4):371–4. https://doi.org/10.1212/CPJ.0000000000000836.
10. Lechien JR, Chiesa-Estomba CM, Cabaraux P, et al. Features of mild-to-moderate COVID-19 patients with dysphonia [published online ahead of print, 2020 Jun 4]. J Voice. 2020;S0892-1997(20)30183–1. https://doi.org/10.1016/j.jvoice.2020.05.012.

11. Li Y, He F, Zhou N, Wei J, Ding Z, Wang L, et al. Organ function support in patients with coronavirus disease 2019: Tongji experience. Front Med. 2020;14(2):232–48. https://doi.org/10.1007/s11684-020-0774-9.
12. Hardin M, Silverman EK. Chronic obstructive pulmonary disease genetics: a review of the past and a look into the future. Chronic Obstr Pulm Dis. 2014;1(1):33–46. https://doi.org/10.15326/jcopdf.1.1.2014.0120.
13. Wada N, Fukunaga K, Obata T, Saito Y, Tamaki H, Kobayashi S, Ka et al. [The respiratory function in children with collagen disease]. Rymachi. 1991;31(5):488–92.
14. Tachikawa R, Tomii K, Ueda H, Nagata K, Nanjo S, Sakurai A, et al. Clinical features and outcome of acute exacerbation of interstitial pneumonia: collagen vascular diseases-related versus idiopathic. Respiration. 2012;83(1):20–7. https://doi.org/10.1159/000329893.
15. Nagao T, Nagai S, Kitaichi M, Hayashi M, Shigematsu M, Tsutsumi T, et al. Usual interstitial pneumonia: idiopathic pulmonary fibrosis versus collagen vascular disease. Respiration. 2001;68(2):151–9. https://doi.org/10.1159/000050485.
16. Richardson AE, Warrier K, Vyas H. Respiratory complication of the rheumatological diseases in childhood. Arch Dis Child. 2016;101(8):752–8. https://doi.org/10.1136/archdischild-2014-306049.
17. Grzywa-Celinska A, Dyczko M, Rekas-Wojcik A, Szmygin-Milanowska K, Witczak A, Ostrowski S, et al. [Ventilatory disorders in patients with chronic heart failure]. Pol Merkur Lekarski. 2015;39(232):248–50.
18. Vitali C, Viegi G, Tassoni S, Tavoni A, Paoletti P, Bibolotti E, et al. Lung function abnormalities in different connective tissue diseases. Clin Rheumatol. 1986;5(2):181–8. https://doi.org/10.1007/BF02032355.
19. Dong X, Zheng Y, Wang L, Chen WH, Zhang YG, Fu Q. Clinical characteristics of autoimmune rheumatic disease-related organizing pneumonia. Clin Rhuematol. 2018;37(4):1027–35. https://doi.org/10.1007/s10067-017-3694-6.
20. Maclean J, Singh RB, Sayeed ZA. Polymyositis presenting with respiratory failure. Indian J Chest Dis Allied Sci. 2011;53(4):229–31.
21. Belafsky PC, Mims JW, Postma GN, Koufman JA. Dysphagia and aspiration secondary to polymyositis. Ear Nose Throat J. 2002;81(5):316.
22. Ji S, Zeng F, Guo Q, Tan G, Tang H, Luo Y, et al. Predictive factors and unfavourable prognostic factors of interstitial lung disease in patients with polymysitis or dermatomyositis: a retrospective study. Chin Med J (Eng). 2010;123(5):517–22.
23. Demoruelle MK, Solomon JJ, Fischer A, Deane KD. The lung may play a role in the pathogenesis of rheumatoid arthritis. Int J Clin Rheumtol. 2014;9(3):295–309. https://doi.org/10.2217/ijr.14.23.
24. Klareskog L, Padyukov L, Ronnelid J, Alfresson L. Genes, environment and immunity in the development of rheumatoid arthritis. Curr Opin Immunol. 2006;18(6):650–5. https://doi.org/10.1016/j.coi.2006.06.004.
25. Klareskog L, Stolt P, Lundberg K, Kallberg H, Bengtsson C, Grunewald J, et al. A new model for an etiology of rheumatoid arthritis: smoking may trigger HLA-DR (shared epitope)-restricted immune reactions to autoantigens modified by citrullination. Arthritis Rheum. 2006;54(1):38/46. https://doi.org/10.1002/art.21575.
26. Steen VD, Conte C, Owens GR, Medsgeer TA. Severe restrictive lung disease in systemic sclerosis. Arthritis Rheum. 1985;37:1283–9. https://doi.org/10.1002/art.1780370903.
27. Solomon JJ, Olson AL, Fischer A, Bull T, Brown KK, Raghu G. Scleroderma lung disease. Eur Respir Rev. 2013;22(127):6–19. https://doi.org/10.1183/09059180.00005512.
28. Tyndall AJ, Bannert B, Vonk M, Airo P, Cozzi F, Carreira PE, et al. Causes and risk factors for death in systemic sclerosis: a study from the EULARR Scleroderma Trials and Research (EUSTAR) database. Ann Rhuem Dis. 2010;69:1809–15. https://doi.org/10.1136/ard.2009.114264.
29. Palm O, Garen T, Berge Enger T, Jensen JL, Lund M-B, Aaløkken TM, et al. Clinical pulmonary involvement in primary Sjogren's syndrome: prevalence, quality of life and mortality—a

retrospective study based on registry data. Rheumatology (Oxford). 2013;52(1):173–9. https:// doi.org/10.1093/rheumatology/kes311.

30. Mavragani CP, Moutsopoulos NM, Moutsopoulos HM. The management of Sjogren's syndrome. Nat Clin Pract Rheumatol. 2006;2(5):252–61. https://doi.org/10.1038/ncprheum0165.

31. Nielepkowicz-Gozdzinska A, Fendler W, Robak E, Kulczycka-Siennicka L, Gorski P, Pietras T, et al. Exhaled IL-8 in systemic lupus erythematosus with and without pulmonary fibrosis. Arch Immunol Ther Exp. 2014;62(3):231–8. https://doi.org/10.1007/s00005-014-0270-5.

32. Fava A, Petri M. Systemic lupus erythematosus: diagnosis and clinical management. Autoimmunity. 2019;96:1–13. https://doi.org/10.1016/j.jaut.2018.11.001.

33. Fortuna G, Brennan MT. Systemic lupus erythematosus: epidemiology, pathophysiology, manifestations, and management. Dent Clin N Am. 2013;57(4):631–55. https://doi.org/10.1016/j. cden.2013.06.003.

34. Alexander FM. The use of self. London: Methuen; 1932.

35. Hoit JD, Hixon TJ. Body type and speech breathing. J Speech Hear Res. 1986;29(3):313–24. https://doi.org/10.1044/jshr.2903.313.

36. Carroll LM. The role of the voice specialist in the non-medical management of benign voice disorders. In: Rubin J, Sataloff RT, Korovin GS, editors. Diagnosis and treatment of voice disorders. 2nd ed. Clifton Park, NY: Delmar Learning; 2003.

37. Mailander E, Muhre L, Barsties B. Lax Vox as a voice training program for teachers: a pilot study. J Voice. 2017;31(2):262.e13–22. https://doi.org/10.1016/j.jvoice.2016.04.011.

38. Guzman M, Laukkanen AM, Krupa P, Horacek J, Svec J, Geneid A. Vocal tract and glottal function during and after vocal exercising with resonance tube and straw. J Voice. 2013;27(4):523. e19–34. https://doi.org/10.1016/j.jvoice.2013.02.007.

Aisha N. Hasan

10.1 Etiologic Agent, Disease Burden, Transmission, and Clinical Course

The outbreak of coronavirus disease 2019 (COVID-19) due to SARS-CoV-2 infection, with initial cases described in China, has now spread to over 180 countries worldwide since January 2020. The World Health Organization (WHO) declared COVID-19 a pandemic on March 11, 2020 [1].

As of April 30th, globally 3,759,967 cases and 259,474 deaths due to COVID 19 have been reported. The US has reported 1,248,040 confirmed cases and 75,477 deaths as of May 8th, and the rates of infection continue to rise in parts of the country.

SARS-CoV-2 is a single stranded RNA virus belonging to the betacoronavirus genus, and has 79% genetic homology to the closely related human coronavirus SARS-CoV, and 98% homology to bat coronavirus RaTG13 [2]. Bats and birds serve as the typical coronavirus hosts, with zoonotic spread and a long-documented history of animal-animal-human transmission [3]. In humans, three pathogenic coronaviruses (severe acute respiratory syndrome coronavirus (SARS-CoV), Middle East respiratory syndrome coronavirus (MERS-CoV) and SARS-CoV-2) can replicate in the lower respiratory tract and cause pneumonia, which can be fatal.

Like the other respiratory coronaviruses, SARS-CoV2 is transmitted primarily via aerosolized respiratory droplets, or direct contact through droplets deposited on surfaces, with a possible, but unproven, fecal–oral transmission route [3].

A. N. Hasan (✉)
Division of Bone Marrow Transplantation, Memorial Sloan Kettering Cancer Center, New York, NY, USA
e-mail: hasana@mskcc.org

10.2 Pathogenesis and Clinical Course

10.2.1 Viral Entry Through Cell Surface ACE-2 Receptor and Predilection for Respiratory Infection

The envelope of the SARS-CoV-2 virus is covered by a surface glycoprotein layer, giving it the characteristic corona appearance on electron microscopy [2]. The peplomers within the glycoprotein layer are known as spike proteins, or S protein, which are likely responsible for the tropism displayed by the virus, as it only engages with specific cell surface receptors; the host cell ACE2 [4]. Previous work on SARS-CoV has established that the virus gains entry into host cells by engaging with the target receptor; the angiotensin-converting enzyme 2 (ACE2). Binding of the virus to a host cell through its target receptor ACE2 is the first step in SARS-Cov2 infection. The virus specifically infects the respiratory tract epithelium since these cells express the target receptor ACE2. The virus enters the airway and alveolar epithelial cells, lung macrophages, and vascular endothelial cells by binding to ACE 2 expressed on the cell surface. SARS-Cov2 is a cytopathic virus which induces death and injury of virus-infected cells as part of the virus replicative cycle [5].

Infection with the SARS-CoV-2 induces an aggressive inflammatory response, which is characterized by release of inflammatory cytokines, elevated acute phase reactants and a cytokine release syndrome (CRS) clinically marked by high fevers, hypoxemia, and hemodynamic instability [6]. This acute inflammation and CRS has been strongly implicated in the resulting damage to the airways [7]. Viral entry activates the targeted resident alveolar macrophages, which then initiates a cascading inflammatory response (Fig. 10.1), that culminates into pathological changes creating ARDS [8]. Activated resident alveolar macrophages leads to release of potent proinflammatory mediators and chemokines which facilitate the accumulation of neutrophils and monocytes. Activated neutrophils further contribute to injury of lung tissue by releasing toxic mediators. The resulting injury disrupts the barrier function of the alveolar epithelium, and also leads to interstitial and intra alveolar flooding. Tumor necrosis factor (TNF)–mediated expression of tissue factor promotes platelet aggregation and microthrombus formation, as well as intraalveolar coagulation and hyaline-membrane formation [8] (Table 10.1).

The degree of inflammation is dependent on the host immune response to viral infection, which determines the severity of respiratory disease.

In addition, after SARS-CoV-2 infection, the ACE 2 expression is reduced in infected lung epithelium. Since loss of pulmonary ACE2 function is associated with acute lung injury, virus-induced ACE2 downregulation may be critical for disease pathology [10].

10.2.2 Role of ACE 2 Expression in Other Vital Organs in Overall Severity of Infection

The ACE2 receptor, which is the main binding site for SARS-CoV-2, is also expressed in the kidney, potentially higher than the lungs [11]. ACE 2 is also

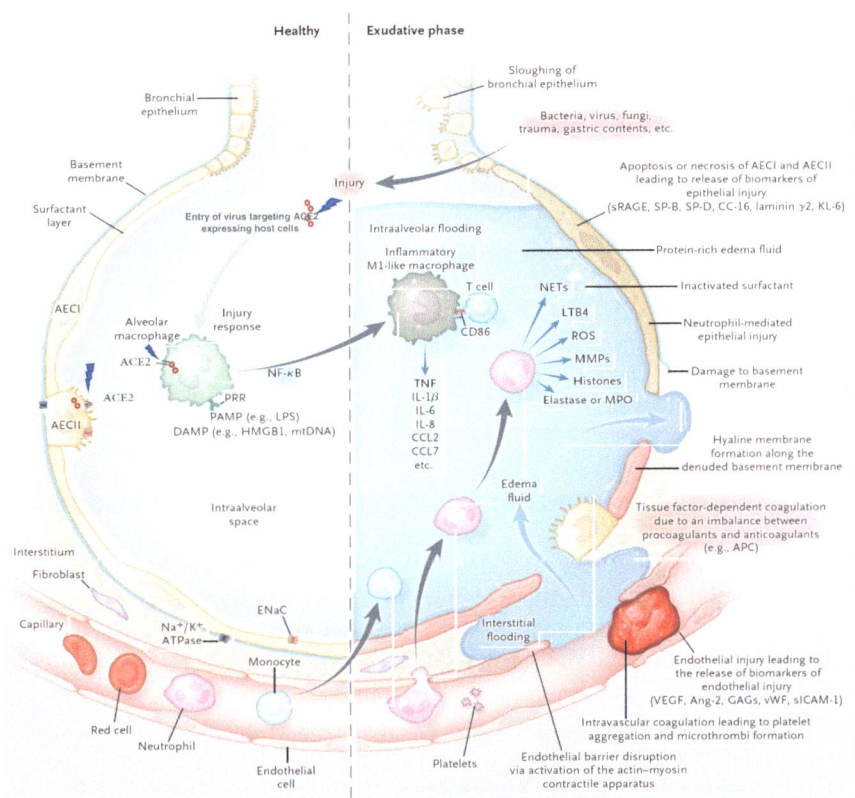

Fig. 10.1 Infection-induced pathogenesis of lung Inflammation and progression to exudative ARDS (L = healthy Lung, R = ARDS). (Adopted from: **B. Taylor Thompson et al. N Engl J Med 2017;377:562–72**)

Table 10.1 Pneumonia severity index (American Thoracic Society) [9]

Minor criteria	Respiratory rate	≥30 breaths/min
	Pa_{O_2} / FI_{O_2}	≤250
	Multilobar infiltrates	✓
	Confusion/disorientation	✓
	Uremia (BUN level)	≥20 mg/dL
	Leukopenia (WBC)	<4000 cells/μL
	Thrombocytopenia (platelet count)	<100,000/μL
	Hypothermia (core temperature)	<36 °C
Major criteria	Hypotension	Requiring aggressive fluid resuscitation
	Septic shock	With need for vasopressors
	Respiratory failure	Requiring mechanical ventilation

involved in regulation of the renin-angiotensin system (RAS). The cytopathic effects instigated by the virus in the kidney tubules, and reduction in ACE2 function after viral infection could result in a dysfunction of the RAS, which can enhance airway inflammation and vascular permeability by influencing blood pressure and fluid/electrolyte balance. Concurrent vascular damage mediated by direct cytopathic viral invasion of the endothelial cells, can further perpetuate and intensify the ongoing inflammatory cascade.

Inflammation resulting from the viral infection can also lead to small vessel microangiopathy that can directly cause myocardial injury that mimics myocardial infarction [12].

Overall, concurrent intra alveolar inflammation, with increased vascular permeability, and increased cardiac preload due to myocardial injury lead to fluid overloaded lungs with severely limited respiratory gas exchange leading to ARDS.

10.2.3 Inflammatory Immunopathogenesis and Coagulopathies

SARS-CoV-2 infection is a cytopathic virus, which triggers an immune response upon invasion into the cell. Although this process is capable of resolving the infection in most cases, an occasional dysfunctional immune response can cause severe respiratory and even systemic pathology. In severe cases, catastrophic outcomes result from an intense surge of systemic immune-inflammation. This highly inflammatory form of programmed cell death due to the cytopathic effects of the virus is called pyroptosis, and when it occurs in lung epithelial cells, the resulting immune response leads to recruitment of macrophages and monocytes, release of cytokines and priming of adaptive T and B cell immune responses [13]. IL-1β, an important cytokine released during pyroptosis, is elevated during SARS-CoV-2 infection.

In a proportion of patients, coagulation abnormalities develop from the profound inflammatory response with SARS-Cov-2 infection. In the early phases of infection, these COVID-19 associated coagulopathies consist of isolated test abnormalities and do not satisfy true criteria of a clinical coagulopathy where impaired ability to clot results in bleeding. The typical abnormalities in early infection include elevated D-dimer and fibrin degradation products, while abnormalities in prothrombin time, partial thromboplastin time, and platelet counts only occur later with further clinical deterioration. In a recent series from china of severely ill ICU patients, factors associated with mortality were increasing D-dimer (>1), lymphopenia, and renal dysfunction, with evidence of DIC [14].

Patients with severe COVID-19 disease admitted to the ICU have been reported to have a higher incidence of venous thromboembolism (VTE) despite standard VTE prophylaxis, compared to historic ICU rates. In a French study of 195 ICU admitted patients with ARDS, there was a significantly higher incidence of life-threatening venous thromboembolism (16.7%) in COVID-19 positive patients compared to non-COVID patients. Among the thrombotic complications, pulmonary embolism was the most commonly observed [15], with an incidence ranging from 11.7% to 20.6% vs. 2.1% to 6.1% in non-COVID patients [16].

10.2.4 End Organ Damage with Evidence of Complement Activation

In severe disease with vascular compromise from microangiopathy, autopsy examinations have demonstrated manifestations of microangiopathy in several organ systems, such as the spleen with splenic infarctions, cardiac muscle, as well as cerebral infarctions.

Recent clinical and autopsy reports of COVID-19 from China and the United States confirm increased clotting and disseminated intravascular coagulation with small vessel thrombosis and pulmonary infarction.

10.2.5 Clinical Symptoms and Signs

The median incubation period for SARS-Cov2 is approximately 4–5 days before evidence of clinical symptoms [2, 17, 18], and the vast majority of symptomatic patients manifest symptoms within 10–12 days of infection [18–20].

Infection with severe acute respiratory syndrome coronavirus 2 (SARS-CoV-2) in humans is associated with a broad spectrum of clinical respiratory syndromes, ranging from mild upper airway symptoms to progressive life-threatening viral pneumonia [19, 20].

Patients with coronavirus disease 2019 (COVID-19) present with clinical symptoms of lower respiratory tract illness with fever, dry cough, and dyspnea. The clinical features in patients confirmed to be infected with SARS-CoV-2 include lower respiratory tract illness with fever, dry cough, and dyspnea [21–23], a manifestation similar to those of two other diseases caused by coronaviruses, severe acute respiratory syndrome (SARS) and Middle East respiratory syndrome (MERS) [24, 25]. Typically at the point of hospital admission, patients may also experience difficulty in breathing, muscle and/or joint pain, headache/dizziness, diarrhea, nausea, and the coughing up of blood [26–28]. Hypoxic respiratory failure and pneumonia coinfection have been the most common acute medical conditions during hospitalization [29]. In severe cases, labored breathing develops with progressive hypoxemia necessitating mechanical ventilatory support. Approximately 20–30% of cases with lower respiratory tract infection, may progress to develop acute respiratory distress syndrome (ARDS) [8], on average around 8–9 days after symptom onset [12, 23]. ARDS in severe COVID-19 disease is characterized by difficulty in breathing with poor alveolar oxygen exchange manifesting as low blood arterial oxygen saturation, progressing to ineffective gas exchange and requiring mechanical ventilation [30].

Some patients may succumb to secondary bacterial and fungal infections. ARDS may also directly cause respiratory failure, which is the cause of death in 70% of fatal COVID-19 cases [29, 30].

The immune response to the viral infection or secondary infection results in massive release of cytokines by the immune system causing a cytokine storm with clinical symptoms of sepsis that are the cause of death in 28% of fatal COVID-19 cases. In such cases, the uncontrolled inflammation cascades into multi- organ damage leading to organ failure, especially of the cardiac, hepatic and renal systems. Majority of SARS-CoV infected patients who progressed to renal failure eventually died [31].

In severe disease with vascular compromise from microangiopathy, patients may present with symptoms of loin pain and hematuria suggesting renal infarction, or with blood in the sputum [16], or symptoms of stroke [14]. The data indicates that elevated D-dimer and low platelet levels are correlated with worse Outcomes [32].

10.3   Clinical Assessment

Initial evaluation of patients is guided by clinical symptoms as well as the index of suspicion for complications based on the known pathophysiology of disease.

In addition to vital signs, a baseline assessment of respiratory status should be performed including oropharyngeal examination, chest examination including auscultation, pulse oximetry, and samples should be obtained for a respiratory viral panel [9].

Frequent laboratory abnormalities with SARS-CoV-2 include leukopenia and thrombocytopenia with elevated levels of creatinine, aminotransaminases, and markers of inflammation [9, 22]. The baseline laboratory evaluation should therefore include a complete blood count with differential, electrolytes, transaminases, LDH, and acute phase reactants such as CRP, ferritin. In sicker patients, a sepsis workup is warranted with blood and sputum cultures as well as venous lactate level and procalcitonin [27, 29]. Inflammatory markers may also be included in the baseline workup including IL-6 (if available) and an ESR to serve as a guide for follow up (see Table 10.2).

10.3.1 Imaging

Radiographic evaluation of the chest is warranted in symptomatic patients. A chest CT should be performed in patients presenting with a high fever suspected to have

Table 10.2 The calculator of CALL points [33]

Comorbidity	
Without	1
With	4
Age (years)	
$\leq$60	1
>60	3
Lymphocyte ($\times 10^9$/L)	
>1.0	1
$\leq$1.0	3
LDH (U/L)	
$\leq$250	1
250–500	2
>500	3

SARS-CoV-2, and in patients with respiratory symptoms and hypoxemia. In the largest reported series of COVID 19 pneumonia [34], all patients had abnormal CT imaging features, and the most common symptoms at onset were fever (73%) and dry cough (59%). Therefore, CT is important in the diagnosis and treatment of COVID-19 pneumonia, and the reported imaging features for this disease are diverse, ranging from normal appearance to diffuse changes in the lungs. Early recognition of the disease is essential for the management of these patients because the time between onset of symptoms and the development of acute respiratory distress syndrome (ARDS) can be as short 8–10 days among the initial patients with COVID-19 pneumonia. In addition, different radiological patterns are observed at different times throughout the disease course.

In order to facilitate early diagnosis of this newly emerging, life-threatening infection Shi et al. analyzed the evolution of chest CT imaging features in patients with COVID-19 pneumonia, and compared the imaging findings across the disease course [34]. Patients were grouped into 4 categories based on the time interval between onset of symptoms and the CT scan: CT scan before symptom onset (group 1); ≤1 week after symptom onset (group 2); >1 to 2 weeks after symptom onset (group 3); and >2 weeks to 3 weeks after symptom onset (group 4). All patients imaged had abnormal CT scans, and although all lung segments can be involved, there was a slight predilection for the right lower lobe. Bilateral lung involvement was observed in 79% of the patients and 44% of patients had diffuse pattern of involvement on scans. The most common patterns seen on chest CT were ground-glass opacities (65%), with ill-defined margins (81%), and importantly, specific CT findings were observed during different phases of disease progression. In the earliest, preclinical stage, CT findings comprised unilateral and multifocal (60%) ground-glass opacification, and rarely included septal or pleural thickening, nodules, cystic changes, pleural effusion, or lymphadenopathy. After the first week of symptom onset, CT lesions progressed to bilateral and diffuse lung involvement, but maintained the appearance of ground-glass opacity. At this stage, pleural effusion and lymphadenopathy could be detected. In the second week, as the disease progressed, the pattern of ground-glass opacity remained the predominant CT finding; however, consolidation patterns were also observed. In the third week after symptom onset, ground-glass opacities and reticular patterns constituted the predominant imaging patterns, while thickening of the adjacent pleura, bronchiectasis, pleural effusions and lymphadenopathy could also be seen at this stage.

Figure 10.2 shows representative CT images of early pulmonary infection (a) and progression of COVID 19 pneumonia (b), (c) and (d).

In terms of laboratory parameters, patients with subclinical pneumonia (group 1) had significantly lower mean concentrations of C-reactive protein (6.9 mg/L, $p = 0.0051$) and aspartate aminotransferase (30.2 U/L, $p = 0.0026$) than patients with clinical manifestations of pneumonia (groups 2–4).

Identifying risk factors at presentation that predict the likelihood of disease progression would help the physicians to decide which group of patients can be managed safely at district hospitals and who needs early transfer to tertiary centers. Age, comorbidities, lymphopenia, serum ferritin, D-dimer levels, cardiac troponin I,

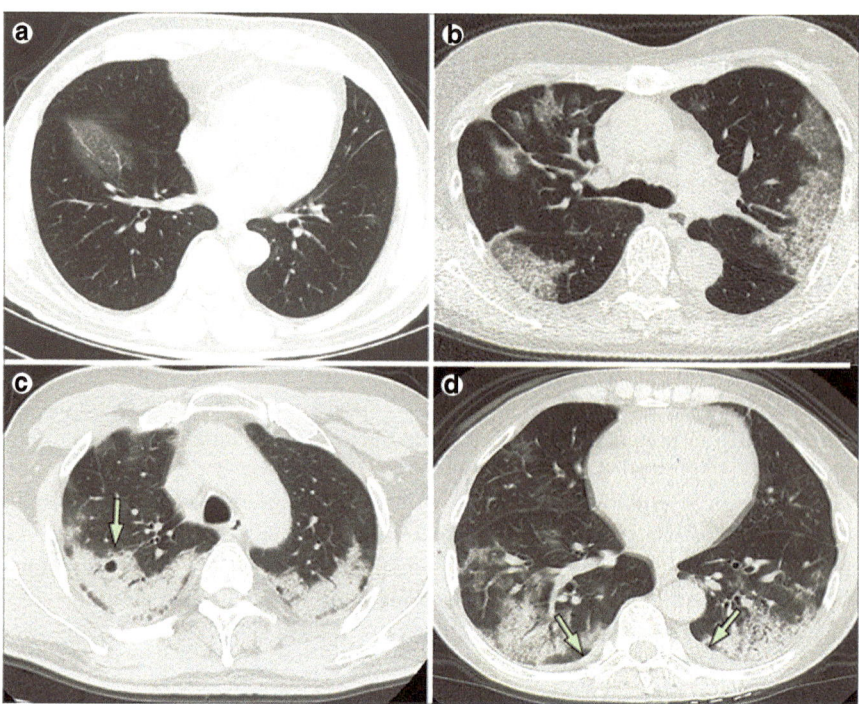

Fig. 10.2 Transverse thin-section CT scans in patients with COVID-19 pneumonia. (**a**) Focal ground-glass opacity associated with septal thickening in the right lower lobes. (**b**) Bilateral, peripheral ground-glass opacity associated with septal thickening (crazy-paving pattern). (**c**) Bilateral and peripheral predominant consolidation pattern with a round cystic change internally (arrow). (**d**) Bilateral, peripheral mixed pattern associated with air bronchograms in both lower and upper lobes, with a small amount of pleural effusion (arrows). (Shi, H et al. ***Lancet Infect Dis 2020;20:425–34***)

lactate dehydrogenase, IL-6, subsets had been shown to be associated with poor prognosis and increased mortalities [22, 35, 36].

Overall, initially, patients with COVID-19 in the ICU develop increased alveolar capillary permeability and subsequent interstitial edema. The presence of edema is illustrated by ground-glass opacities of the lung parenchyma on lung CT. Postmortem examination of patients with COVID 19 pneumonia, showed patchy involvement of the lungs on macroscopic examination, with congested and edematous lungs. Histological examination further revealed features suggestive of exudative and early or intermediate proliferative phases of diffuse alveolar damage (Fig. 10.3), with focal patterns of interstitial pneumonia (inflammatory lymphomonocytic infiltrate alongside thickened interalveolar septa), organizing pneumonia (alveolar loose plugs of fibroblastic tissue), and acute fibrinous organizing pneumonia (some alveolar spaces containing granulocytes and fibrin) [37]. Strikingly, there has not been any evidence of fibrotic phase of diffuse alveolar damage, such as mural fibrosis and microcystic honeycombing,

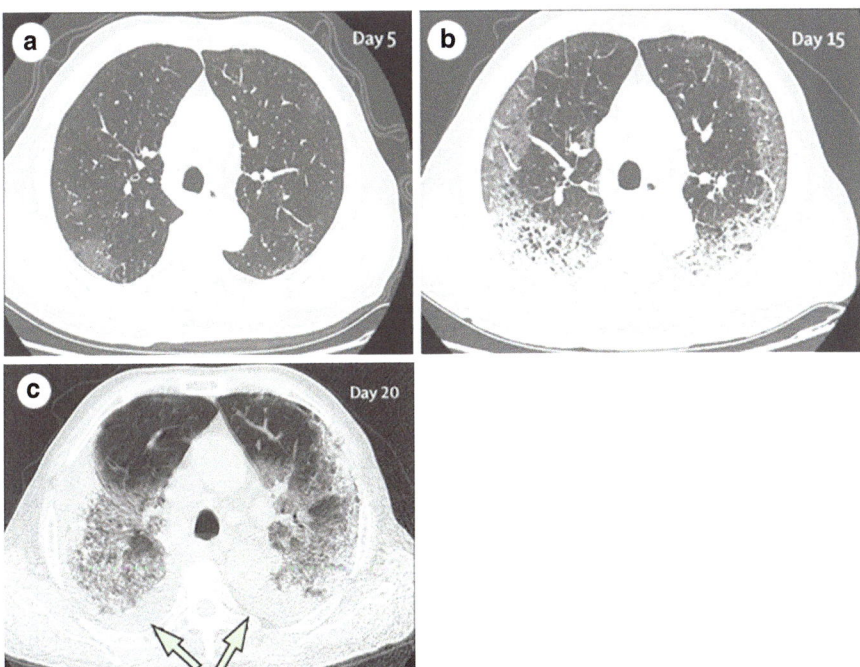

Fig. 10.3 Progression of COVID-19 Pneumonia. (**a**) Day 5 after symptom onset: patchy ground-glass opacities affecting the bilateral, subpleural lung parenchyma. (**b**) Day 15: subpleural crescent-shaped ground-glass opacities in both lungs, as well as posterior reticular opacities and subpleural crescent-shaped consolidations. (**c**) Day 20: expansion of bilateral pulmonary lesions, with enlargement and denser pulmonary consolidations and bilateral pleural effusions (arrows). The patient died 10 days after the final scan. (Shi, H et al. *Lancet Infect Dis* **2020;20:425–34**)

suggesting that patients typically do not progress to the fibrotic phase, possibly because of the short duration of the disease compared to long standing COPD or BOOP.

If patients require mechanical ventilation, oxygenation improves following prone positioning, higher PEEP, and restrictive fluid management. Subsequently, their condition might deteriorate suddenly, and pulmonary embolism can occur, detected by contrast-enhanced lung CT scan.

A retrospective analysis of 208 consecutive patients at 2 Chinese centers, elucidated 4 key factors predictive of disease severity, including age, lymphocyte count, comorbidities, and serum LDH. A score of 10–13 points had greater than 50% probability of severe disease. Although these data need prospective validation in larger patient populations, it serves as a screening tool for initial risk assessment for guiding clinical management [33].

In patients who develop disease, assessment of complications allows for prediction of outcome. The sequential organ failure assessment score (SOFA) is a prognostic tool used in the ICU setting [38]. In assessing risk factors contributing to in hospital death for patients with severe COVID-19 disease, an increasing odds of

Table 10.3 The Sequential Organ Failure Assessment Score (SOFA)

Variables		0	1	2	3	4
Respiratory	Pao$_2$/Fio$_2$ mmHg	>400	≤400	≤300	≤200[a]	≤100[a]
Coagulation	Platelets × 10^3	>150	≤150	≤100	≤50	≤20
Liver	Bilirubin, mg/dL	<1.2	1.2–1.9	2.0–5.9	6.0–11.9	>12.0
Cardiovascular	Hypotension	No	MAP < 70 mmHg	Dop ≤ or Dob (any dose)[b]	Dop > 5; Epi ≤ 0.1; or Nor epi ≤ 0.1[b]	Dop > 15; Epi > 0.1; or Nor epi > 0.1[b]
Central Nervous System	Glasgow Coma Score Scale	15	13–14	10–12	6–9	<6
Renal	Creatinine, mg/dL or urine output, mL/dL	<1.2	1.2–1.9	2.0–3.4	3.5–4.9 or <500	>5.0 or <200

[a]Values are with respiratory support
[b]Adrenergic agents administered for at least 1 h (doses in μg/kg/min)

death was associated with older age, higher SOFA score, and D-dimer >1 μg/mL at the time of admission [12] (Table 10.3).

10.3.2 Therapies Under Evaluation for Managing Severe COVID-19 Disease

Insights gained from initial cases, including autopsy findings have been instrumental in understanding mechanisms responsible for the severe clinical course in this disease. The recognition of the rapidly escalating burden of infection, and rising death rates have galvanized efforts toward rapid initiation of clinical trials. A search for COVID-19-related clinical trials on clinicaltrials.gov as of May 11th, identified 1358 studies worldwide, of which 808 were interventional studies. The list is exhaustive including novel agents as well as agents addressing pathogenesis of disease. The major pathology caused by viral infection is damage to the respiratory/ lung epithelium and inflammatory surge. Clinical assessment and management of patients presenting with pneumonia is guided by symptom severity guided by the ATS symptom score in Table 10.2.

Patients with lung disease are typically treated with broad-spectrum antibiotics, inhaled bronchodilators, and/or systemic steroids.

For symptomatic management of severe illness, respiratory support should be provided with prone positioning, supplemental oxygen and mechanical ventilation. Because the virus can infect monocytes and macrophages and cause aberrant cytokine secretion, the resulting systemic inflammation is treated with immune modulating agents such as systemic steroids such as dexamethasone [39], anti-IL-6 R (tocilizumab), anti-IL-1β (anakinra).

In view of the adverse outcomes with development of coagulopathies, prophylactic anticoagulants have been administered to patients with disease. Prophylactic doses of heparin in patients with D-dimer exceeding 3.0 µg/mL demonstrated a 20% reduction in mortality (32.8% vs. 52.4%, $p = 0.017$) [40].

In addition, antiviral agents including neutralizing antibodies are being investigated for their therapeutic potential. The antiviral agent remdesivir has demonstrated clinical benefit in patients with severe COVID 19 disease, and has been recently FDA approved for treatment of infected patients. In addition to remdesivir, other antivirals are also being used empirically for treatment.

In critically ill patients in the ICU, convalescent donor plasma is also being administered though the specific clinical benefit of this therapeutic modality has not been fully characterized in this disease.

10.4 Clinical Perspective on Available Data

The pandemic of SARS-CoV-2 is a historic event in modern times that is sure to reset norms. The abruptly imposed social distancing in an era embedded in social media, a society habituated to packed interactive schedules, cosmetic treatments and record high international travel, has disrupted life for the near term. The medical scientific community has demonstrated extraordinary innovative abilities in rapid initiation of clinical trials to overcome this gigantic health care crisis. In addition to developing novel agents, previously known agents used in other indications have been repurposed and applied to treatment of COVID-19 disease for management of various associated clinical symptoms. For example, Tocilizumab, an IL-6 receptor antagonist, is an anti-inflammatory agent that is approved for the treatment of rheumatoid arthritis, and also for the treatment of severe cytokine release syndrome (CRS) associated with CAR engineered T-cell therapies for cancer [41]. Its distinct efficacy in controlling CRS, was leveraged to enable use for severely ill COVID-19 infected patients. Similar innovations include the use of hydroxochloroquine and Ivermectin, which are both anti-parasitic agents, and the former also anti-inflammatory, however, experimental observations of activity against the virus permitted initial clinical investigations.

In view of the poor outcomes of patients who develop ARDS, measures such as use of surfactant (typically used in preterm babies with hyaline-membrane disease), nitric oxide and high frequency ventilation, are all innovative approaches for managing critically ill patients with this disease and enable survival.

On the technology side, novel approaches for infection tracking have been put in place using machine learning to estimate unobserved COVID-19 infections in North America [42].

In anticipation of an effective vaccine, and reliable testing methods, the medical community is focused on collecting data with the tested approaches. In the next few months, maturing data emerging from controlled trials will help consolidate treatment algorithms that will improve outcomes with COVID-19 disease.

References

1. World Health Organization. Virtual press conference on Covid-19. 11 March 2020. https://www.who.int/docs/default-source/coronaviruse/transcripts/who-audio-emergencies-coronavirus-press-conference-full-and-final-11mar2020.pdf?sfvrsn=cb432bb3_2. Accessed 23 Feb 2021.
2. Coronaviridae Study Group of the International Committee on Taxonomy of V. The species severe acute respiratory syndrome-related coronavirus: classifying 2019-nCoV and naming it SARS-CoV-2. Nat Microbiol. 2020;5(4):536–44. https://doi.org/10.1038/s41564-020-0695-z.
3. Zhou P, Yang XL, Wang XG, Hu B, Zhang L, Zhang W, et al. A pneumonia outbreak associated with a new coronavirus of probable bat origin. Nature. 2020;579(7798):270–3. https://doi.org/10.1038/s41586-020-2012-7.
4. Walls AC, Park YJ, Tortorici MA, Wall A, McGuire AT, Veesler D. Structure, function, and antigenicity of the SARS-CoV-2 spike glycoprotein. Cell. 2020;181(2):281–92 e6. https://doi.org/10.1016/j.cell.2020.02.058.
5. Park WB, Kwon NJ, Choi SJ, Kang CK, Choe PG, Kim JY, et al. Virus isolation from the first patient with SARS-CoV-2 in Korea. J Korean Med Sci. 2020;35(7):e84. https://doi.org/10.3346/jkms.2020.35.e84.
6. Wang W, Liu X, Wu S, Chen S, Li Y, Nong L, et al. Definition and risks of cytokine release syndrome in 11 critically Ill COVID-19 patients with pneumonia: analysis of disease characteristics. J Infect Dis. 2020;222(9):1444–51. https://doi.org/10.1093/infdis/jiaa387.
7. Wong CK, Lam CW, Wu AK, Ip WK, Lee NL, Chan IH, et al. Plasma inflammatory cytokines and chemokines in severe acute respiratory syndrome. Clin Exp Immunol. 2004;136(1):95–103. https://doi.org/10.1111/j.1365-2249.2004.02415.x.
8. Thompson BT, Chambers RC, Liu KD. Acute respiratory distress syndrome. N Engl J Med. 2017;377(6):562–72. https://doi.org/10.1056/NEJMra1608077.
9. Metlay JP, Waterer GW, Long AC, Anzueto A, Brozek J, Crothers K, et al. Diagnosis and treatment of adults with community-acquired pneumonia. An official clinical practice guideline of the American Thoracic Society and Infectious Diseases Society of America. Am J Respir Crit Care Med. 2019;200(7):e45–67. https://doi.org/10.1164/rccm.201908-1581ST.
10. Imai Y, Kuba K, Rao S, Huan Y, Guo F, Guan B, et al. Angiotensin-converting enzyme 2 protects from severe acute lung failure. Nature. 2005;436(7047):112–6. https://doi.org/10.1038/nature03712.
11. Jia HP, Look DC, Shi L, Hickey M, Pewe L, Netland J, et al. ACE2 receptor expression and severe acute respiratory syndrome coronavirus infection depend on differentiation of human airway epithelia. J Virol. 2005;79(23):14614–21. https://doi.org/10.1128/JVI.79.23.14614-14621.2005.
12. Zhou F, Yu T, Du R, Fan G, Liu Y, Liu Z, et al. Clinical course and risk factors for mortality of adult inpatients with COVID-19 in Wuhan, China: a retrospective cohort study. Lancet. 2020;395(10229):1054–62. https://doi.org/10.1016/S0140-6736(20)30566-3.
13. Zheng M, Williams EP, Malireddi RKS, Karki R, Banoth B, Burton A, et al. Impaired NLRP3 inflammasome activation/pyroptosis leads to robust inflammatory cell death via caspase-8/RIPK3 during coronavirus infection. J Biol Chem. 2020;295(41):14040–52. https://doi.org/10.1074/jbc.RA120.015036.
14. Connors JM, Levy JH. COVID-19 and its implications for thrombosis and anticoagulation. Blood. 2020;135(23):2033–40. https://doi.org/10.1182/blood.2020006000.
15. Helms J, Tacquard C, Severac F, Leonard-Lorant I, Ohana M, Delabranche X, et al. High risk of thrombosis in patients with severe SARS-CoV-2 infection: a multicenter prospective cohort study. Intensive Care Med. 2020;46(6):1089–98. https://doi.org/10.1007/s00134-020-06062-x.
16. Poissy J, Goutay J, Caplan M, Parmentier E, Duburcq T, Lassalle F, et al. Pulmonary embolism in patients with COVID-19: awareness of an increased prevalence. Circulation. 2020;142(2):184–6. https://doi.org/10.1161/CIRCULATIONAHA.120.047430.

17. Guan WJ, Ni ZY, Hu Y, Liang WH, Ou CQ, He JX, et al. Clinical characteristics of corona-virus disease 2019 in China. N Engl J Med. 2020;382(18):1708–20. https://doi.org/10.1056/NEJMoa2002032.
18. Lauer SA, Grantz KH, Bi Q, Jones FK, Zheng Q, Meredith HR, et al. The incubation period of coronavirus disease 2019 (COVID-19) from publicly reported confirmed cases: estimation and application. Ann Intern Med. 2020;172(9):577–82. https://doi.org/10.7326/M20-0504.
19. Chen N, Zhou M, Dong X, Qu J, Gong F, Han Y, et al. Epidemiological and clinical character-istics of 99 cases of 2019 novel coronavirus pneumonia in Wuhan, China: a descriptive study. Lancet. 2020;395(10223):507–13. https://doi.org/10.1016/S0140-6736(20)30211-7.
20. Zhu N, Zhang D, Wang W, Li X, Yang B, Song J, et al. A novel coronavirus from patients with pneumonia in China, 2019. N Engl J Med. 2020;382(8):727–33. https://doi.org/10.1056/NEJMoa2001017.
21. Grasselli G, Zangrillo A, Zanella A, Antonelli M, Cabrini L, Castelli A, et al. Baseline char-acteristics and outcomes of 1591 patients infected with SARS-CoV-2 admitted to ICUs of the Lombardy Region, Italy. JAMA. 2020;323(16):1574–81. https://doi.org/10.1001/jama.2020.5394.
22. Huang C, Wang Y, Li X, Ren L, Zhao J, Hu Y, et al. Clinical features of patients infected with 2019 novel coronavirus in Wuhan, China. Lancet. 2020;395(10223):497–506. https://doi.org/10.1016/S0140-6736(20)30183-5.
23. Richardson S, Hirsch JS, Narasimhan M, Crawford JM, McGinn T, Davidson KW, et al. Presenting characteristics, comorbidities, and outcomes among 5700 patients hospitalized with COVID-19 in the New York City Area. JAMA. 2020;323(20):2052–9. https://doi.org/10.1001/jama.2020.6775.
24. Assiri A, Al-Tawfiq JA, Al-Rabeeah AA, Al-Rabiah FA, Al-Hajjar S, Al-Barrak A, et al. Epidemiological, demographic, and clinical characteristics of 47 cases of Middle East respira-tory syndrome coronavirus disease from Saudi Arabia: a descriptive study. Lancet Infect Dis. 2013;13(9):752–61. https://doi.org/10.1016/S1473-3099(13)70204-4.
25. Tsang KW, Ho PL, Ooi GC, Yee WK, Wang T, Chan-Yeung M, et al. A cluster of cases of severe acute respiratory syndrome in Hong Kong. N Engl J Med. 2003;348(20):1977–85. https://doi.org/10.1056/NEJMoa030666.
26. Chan JF, Yuan S, Kok KH, To KK, Chu H, Yang J, et al. A familial cluster of pneumonia associated with the 2019 novel coronavirus indicating person-to-person transmission: a study of a family cluster. Lancet. 2020;395(10223):514–23. https://doi.org/10.1016/S0140-6736(20)30154-9.
27. Chen G, Wu D, Guo W, Cao Y, Huang D, Wang H, et al. Clinical and immunological features of severe and moderate coronavirus disease 2019. J Clin Invest. 2020;130(5):2620–9. https://doi.org/10.1172/JCI137244.
28. Li Q, Guan X, Wu P, Wang X, Zhou L, Tong Y, et al. Early transmission dynamics in Wuhan, China, of novel coronavirus-infected pneumonia. N Engl J Med. 2020;382(13):1199–207. https://doi.org/10.1056/NEJMoa2001316.
29. Price-Haywood EG, Burton J, Fort D, Seoane L. Hospitalization and mortality among black patients and white patients with covid-19. N Engl J Med. 2020;382(26):2534–43. https://doi.org/10.1056/NEJMsa2011686.
30. Zhang B, Zhou X, Qiu Y, Song Y, Feng F, Feng J, et al. Clinical characteristics of 82 cases of death from COVID-19. PLoS One. 2020;15(7):e0235458. https://doi.org/10.1371/journal.pone.0235458.
31. Chu KH, Tsang WK, Tang CS, Lam MF, Lai FM, To KF, et al. Acute renal impairment in coronavirus-associated severe acute respiratory syndrome. Kidney Int. 2005;67(2):698–705. https://doi.org/10.1111/j.1523-1755.2005.67130.x.
32. Tang N, Li D, Wang X, Sun Z. Abnormal coagulation parameters are associated with poor prog-nosis in patients with novel coronavirus pneumonia. J Thromb Haemost. 2020;18(4):844–7. https://doi.org/10.1111/jth.14768.

33. Ji D, Zhang D, Xu J, Chen Z, Yang T, Zhao P, et al. Prediction for progression risk in patients with COVID-19 pneumonia: the CALL score. Clin Infect Dis. 2020;71(6):1393–9. https://doi.org/10.1093/cid/ciaa414.

34. Shi H, Han X, Jiang N, Cao Y, Alwalid O, Gu J, et al. Radiological findings from 81 patients with COVID-19 pneumonia in Wuhan, China: a descriptive study. Lancet Infect Dis. 2020;20(4):425–34. https://doi.org/10.1016/S1473-3099(20)30086-4.

35. Wang D, Hu B, Hu C, Zhu F, Liu X, Zhang J, et al. Clinical characteristics of 138 hospitalized patients with 2019 novel coronavirus-infected pneumonia in Wuhan, China. JAMA. 2020;323(11):1061–9. https://doi.org/10.1001/jama.2020.1585.

36. Yang X, Yu Y, Xu J, Shu H, Xia J, Liu H, et al. Clinical course and outcomes of critically ill patients with SARS-CoV-2 pneumonia in Wuhan, China: a single-centered, retrospective, observational study. Lancet Respir Med. 2020;8(5):475–81. https://doi.org/10.1016/S2213-2600(20)30079-5.

37. Carsana L, Sonzogni A, Nasr A, Rossi RS, Pellegrinelli A, Zerbi P, et al. Pulmonary post-mortem findings in a series of COVID-19 cases from northern Italy: a two-centre descriptive study. Lancet Infect Dis. 2020;20(10):1135–40. https://doi.org/10.1016/S1473-3099(20)30434-5.

38. Ferreira FL, Bota DP, Bross A, Melot C, Vincent JL. Serial evaluation of the SOFA score to predict outcome in critically ill patients. JAMA. 2001;286(14):1754–8. https://doi.org/10.1001/jama.286.14.1754.

39. Horby P, Lim WS, Emberson JR, Mafham M, Bell JL, Linsell L, et al. Dexamethasone in hospitalized patients with covid-19—preliminary report. N Engl J Med. 2021;384(8):693–704. https://doi.org/10.1056/NEJMoa2021436.

40. Tang N, Bai H, Chen X, Gong J, Li D, Sun Z. Anticoagulant treatment is associated with decreased mortality in severe coronavirus disease 2019 patients with coagulopathy. J Thromb Haemost. 2020;18(5):1094–9. https://doi.org/10.1111/jth.14817.

41. Neelapu SS, Tummala S, Kebriaei P, Wierda W, Gutierrez C, Locke FL, et al. Chimeric antigen receptor T-cell therapy—assessment and management of toxicities. Nat Rev Clin Oncol. 2018;15(1):47–62. https://doi.org/10.1038/nrclinonc.2017.148.

42. Vaid S, Cakan C, Bhandari M. Using machine learning to estimate unobserved COVID-19 infections in North America. J Bone Joint Surg Am. 2020;102(13):e70. https://doi.org/10.2106/JBJS.20.00715.